'Dr Music is certainly one of the best and probably ... psychotherapists in the world. This beautiful book distills decades of neuro-clinical thinking, interpreting children's and young people's experience and behavior in terms of the most applicable and scientifically credible models of mind. For those who wish to understand clinical phenomena and through this improve their clinical work, this book is a must. For those who want to marvel and learn from the writing of a master clinician, this book is amongst the best you are likely to encounter. And for the few who want to do both... this is an incredible opportunity. I could not recommend a book more strongly.'

– Professor Peter Fonagy OBE, Head of the Division of Psychology and Language Sciences at UCL; Chief Executive of the Anna Freud National Centre for Children and Families, London, UK

'Of all life forms on this planet human infants are by far the most dependent on the love and care they receive from their parents. The need for caring can extend well into the adolescent years and beyond. Not only do parents protect them but they shape the maturation of their brain development, the robustness of their immune system and even the expression of their genes. As an international, leading exponent of attachment theory and its applications in child psychotherapy there could be no better guide than Dr Music to reveal the role of attachment as both a source of trauma and its recovery. Bringing the reader many years of therapeutic insight and experience, with a clarity of exposition of fascinating and important case studies, this is a wonderful addition to the literature. All therapists and other professionals working with children would benefit enormously from this book.'

– Professor Paul Gilbert OBE, author of *The Compassionate Mind* and *Living like Crazy*

'Graham Music has done it again. This is a much-needed book and the clinical work is profoundly moving. Music is able to blend his own deeply felt empathic capacities with a comprehensive grasp of the latest developmental and neuroscientific research in a highly readable form. He is a real thinker and all of us in the field of child mental health, and for that matter, learning disability, will be extremely grateful for it. He really gets, and uses, all the new work on the body, too.'

– Anne Alvarez, consultant, child and adolescent psychotherapist, Tavistock Clinic; author of *Live Company* and *The Thinking Heart*

'If you are looking for a book that tells you what attachment-based, neuroscience-informed psychotherapy looks like in practice, look no further. Graham Music's wonderful book conveys the process brilliantly. It demonstrates how an attuned and compassionate relationship is the key to psychological growth, a process that might sound easy yet is in practice a demanding art that draws on all the psychotherapist's resources to respond at the right level, at the right moment. He is particularly good on the psychotherapist's own struggles to extend compassion to himself and to stay "alive and present" in difficult therapeutic relationships.'

– Sue Gerhardt, psychotherapist; co-founder of the Oxford Parent Infant Project; and author of the bestselling book *Why Love Matters*

'Graham Music takes us on a journey with him in his new book, *Nuturing Children: From Trauma to Growth Using Attachment Theory, Psychoanalysis and Neurobiology.* From his psychoanalytic "bedrock" Graham grows flowers, many of which include his reflections on the thoughts of therapeutic mentors and theorists as well as on therapeutic implications from findings of attachment and neurobiology research. Yet the most vibrant flowers involve the moments that he spends coming to know the minds and hearts of young people and discovering the paths with them that will lead from trauma to hope. In this work Graham invites us into his therapeutic space to be present with him – with both his mind and heart – as he is present with these hurt and courageous young people.

To read this work is to enter into a conversation with Graham, to wonder with him about the meanings of what Molly, Michael, Samantha and the others are doing so to better understand their unique experiences and find the one-of-a-kind therapeutic intervention that will do them the most good. We share with Graham his wobbles and confusion, recoveries and unfoldings, as he finds a way of relating with each child that may well create safety, healing, and integration. These conversations, readily available to us as we read, will bring Graham with us into our therapeutic space and enrich our work with the minds and hearts of the children we are coming to know and care about, regardless of the nature of the bedrock upon which we stand.'

– Daniel A. Hughes, PhD, is a clinical psychologist who specializes in child abuse and neglect, attachment, foster care, and adoption. He is a prolific author and actively trains other therapists in the model of treatment known as Dyadic Developmental Psychotherapy, both within the United States and in other countries

Nurturing Children

Nurturing Children describes children's lives transformed through therapy.

Drawing on decades of experience, internationally respected clinician and trainer Graham Music tackles major issues affecting troubled children, including trauma, neglect, depression and violence. Using psychoanalysis alongside modern developmental thinking from neurobiology, attachment and trauma theory and mindfulness, Music creates his own distinctive blend of approaches to help even the most traumatised of children.

A mix of personal accounts and therapeutic riches, *Nurturing Children* will appeal to anyone helping children, young people and families to lead fuller lives.

Graham Music is a consultant child and adolescent psychotherapist at the Tavistock and Portman Clinics in London, UK, and an adult psychotherapist in private practice who teaches, supervises and lectures internationally.

Nurturing Children

From Trauma to Growth Using Attachment Theory, Psychoanalysis and Neurobiology

Graham Music

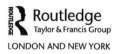
Routledge
Taylor & Francis Group

LONDON AND NEW YORK

First published 2019
by Routledge
2 Park Square, Milton Park, Abingdon, Oxon OX14 4RN

and by Routledge
52 Vanderbilt Avenue, New York, NY 10017

Routledge is an imprint of the Taylor & Francis Group, an informa business

British Library Cataloguing-in-Publication Data
A catalogue record for this book is available from the British Library

Library of Congress Cataloging-in-Publication Data
Names: Music, Graham, 1957- author.
Title: Nurturing children : from trauma to growth using attachment theory, psychoanalysis and neurobiology / Graham Music.
Description: Abingdon, Oxon ; New York, NY : Routledge, 2019.
Identifiers: LCCN 2018039399 (print) | LCCN 2018050323 (ebook) | ISBN 9780429437540 (Master eBook) | ISBN 9780429794360 (Adobe Reader) | ISBN 9780429794353 (ePub) | ISBN 9780429794346 (Mobipocket) | ISBN 9781138346055 | ISBN 9781138346055q(hardback) | ISBN 9781138346062(pbk.) | ISBN 9780429437540(ebook)
Subjects: LCSH: Child psychotherapy. | Adolescent psychotherapy.
Classification: LCC RJ504 (ebook) | LCC RJ504 .M88 2019 (print) | DDC 618.92/8914–dc23
LC record available at https://lccn.loc.gov/2018039399

ISBN: 978-1-138-34605-5 (hbk)
ISBN: 978-1-138-34606-2 (pbk)
ISBN: 978-0-429-43754-0 (ebk)

Typeset in Times New Roman
by Swales & Willis Ltd

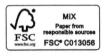

Printed and bound in Great Britain by
TJ International Ltd, Padstow, Cornwall

This book is dedicated to my therapists, Roger, Mike, Celia and Nathan, for facilitating my own journey from trauma and anxiety into more well-being and a Good Life.

Contents

Acknowledgements

I would like to thank the following for reading drafts or chapters, or discussing ideas in this book. Of course, they are in no way responsible for the outcome but I am hugely grateful for their generous help and thoughtfulness: Sue Beecraft, Jed Cameron, Geraldine Crehan, Ricky Emanuel, Sue Gerhardt, Rob Glanz, Paul Gordon, Simon Lynne, Jane O'Rourke, Roz Read, Di Sofer, Peter Speier, Karen Treisman and Helen Wright.

A special thanks also to Lawrence Dodgson for the use of his 'window of tolerance' illustration, and also for the generosity of the International Center for Compassionate Organizations for use of the three-circles model image (Figure 9.2). Thanks also to Becky Hall for permission to use her clinical work.

I am as always indebted to my family, especially Sue and Rose, and also my many good friends, who have sustained me and also put up with my physical and emotional absences while writing this book. I am particularly grateful to my clients and patients who over the years have shown courage in facing complex issues and finding a way to come through stronger and more able to live rich and full lives.

In terms of the stories and clinical accounts in this book, I have maintained strict confidentiality to the best of my knowledge and ability and ensured that client information is non-identifiable. I have of course sought permission to use the material wherever possible. In some cases, strong disguise is used to ensure that specific individuals cannot be recognised, while always trying to remain as true as I could to the emotional truth of the encounters described and the lessons to be learnt from these meetings.

I would like to acknowledge the generosity of the following journals where extracts from some of the chapters were initially published:

Extracts from Chapter 1 were previously published in Music, G. (2004) The old one–two. *Journal of Child Psychotherapy*, 30 (1), pp. 21–37.

Extracts from Chapter 2 were previously published in Music, G. (2005) Surfacing the depths: Thoughts on imitation, resonance and growth. *Journal of Child Psychotherapy*, 31 (1), pp. 72–90.

Extracts from Chapter 5 were previously published in Music, G. (2014) Top down and bottom up: Trauma, executive functioning, emotional-regulation, the brain and child psychotherapy. *Journal of Child Psychotherapy*, 40 (1), pp. 3–19.

Extracts from Chapter 7 were previously published in Music, G. (2009) Neglecting neglect: Some thoughts about children who have lacked good input, and are 'undrawn' and 'unenjoyed'. *Journal of Child Psychotherapy*, 35 (2), pp. 142–156.

Extracts from Chapter 8 were previously published in Music, G. (2015) Bringing up the bodies: Psyche-soma, body awareness and feeling at ease. *British Journal of Psychotherapy*, 31 (1), pp. 4–19.

Extracts from Chapter 10 were previously published in Music, G. (2016) Angels and devils: Sadism and violence in children. *Journal of Child Psychotherapy*, 42 (3), pp. 302–317.

Extracts from Chapter 11 were previously published in Music, G. (2012) Selfless genes, altruism and trauma: Research and clinical implications. *British Journal of Psychotherapy*, 28 (2), pp. 154–171.

Extracts from Chapter 12 were previously published in Music, G. (2014) The buzz trap: Speeded-up lives, distractedness, impulsiveness and decreasing empathy. *Psychodynamic Practice*, 20 (3), pp. 228–249.

Extracts from Chapter 13 were previously published in Music, G. (2008) From scapegoating to thinking and finding a home: Delivering therapeutic work in schools. *Journal of Child Psychotherapy*, 34 (1), pp. 43–61.

Chapter I

Introduction

This book distils key ingredients needed to help emotionally troubled children and young people. Growth, change, well-being and a Good Life spring from having our feelings understood, from experiencing rewarding human relationships and being held in the minds and hearts of others. The stories in this volume make the case for the curative potential of growth-inducing human relationships.

This might sound obvious, but is counter-cultural in a climate emphasising short-term treatments, evidence-based practice and quick-fix ideologies. The evidence for so-called evidenced-based treatment is at best shaky (Shedler, 2018). Most such modalities eschew a commitment to deep interpersonal meetings, to the bearing of difficult thoughts and feelings and to biding one's time. The latest developmental, neurobiological and attachment research, the riches from psychoanalysis and systemic thinking, alongside decades of clinical experience, suggest another, more relationship-based explanation of how change takes place. This is seen in forthcoming chapters where real stories of children and young people take centre stage.

I have worked as a psychotherapist for over three decades with children, young people, families, parents and adults. In such work our learning never ends, even if yesterday's and today's certainty become tomorrow's naive belief. I have often witnessed how psychological shifts take root and how, despite unexpected twists and turns, the capacity to heal and grow can be tapped into. I hope the stories in this book illustrate this.

In my therapeutic life, an extraordinary group of teachers, supervisors and therapists have helped me to find my own way to be a therapist. I have worked in internationally renowned institutions, such as the Tavistock Centre, the Anna Freud Centre, the Portman Clinic and the Centre for

Child Mental Health, and have trained with and worked alongside some of the most eminent in the business. More importantly, I have plied my trade for years in an ordinary way, in community child mental health services, schools, GP practices, specialist adolescent therapy teams and many other settings. Here is where the real learning takes place, via being immersed over time in the lives of those we work with.

I am continually excited about the possibilities that this work affords. We have unendingly interesting ways of understanding children's development, what goes awry, how and why resilience and hope grow, what we can and can't do to restore more positive life trajectories. When my work goes well it is minimally due to my theories and learning, but mainly due to making meaningful, compassionate emotional contact with complex states of mind and feelings in myself and others.

Like anyone trying to help troubled kids, I often feel despondent about what is possible. The unthinkable experiences of some children, their awful life circumstances, the ways we as professionals and society have let them down, can be unbearably painful to face. It is often agonising to confront the horrors of their minds, often filled with aggressive, destructive and nihilistic thoughts and wishes. Perhaps worse, it is excruciating when traumatic experiences lead to self-destructive patterns, lives lived in distrust, hopelessness, rancour and bitterness, with too little self-belief, hope or pleasure.

I believe we are on the cusp of a paradigm shift in therapeutic work, one requiring an integration of multiple orientations, from neurobiology, attachment theory, psychoanalysis, systemic thinking and more. The result of such integration is a fascinating if constantly developing set of new insights. Being open to new ideas requires courage and humility, alongside interest and curiosity. Above all, our work demands a passion, a sense of vocation, and a wish to continually learn, about ourselves, about those who come through our door, new scientific and clinical findings and indeed about life. The fourteenth-century Persian Sufi poet, Hafiz, cautioned against the small-minded building of cages that restrict thinking and urged that we should drop keys to free 'the beautiful rowdy prisoners'. I too want to pass around some of the keys that my heroes of yesteryear generously dropped for us, keys that can unlock the doors to growth and freedom, for both ourselves and those we work with.

Empathy and feeling understood

I try in this book to return to the basics of therapeutic work, what really makes a difference to those in distress. Evidence suggests that the therapeutic alliance is the *sine qua non* of successful therapy, and I unpick some of what this means. Central to transformative relationships are empathy and compassion, making emotional contact with another, showing that we are prepared to join them on a journey, but not as too distant an expert, nor as a fellow traveller lost without a map.

I learnt important lessons about this from delivering non-directive play therapy over 30 years ago, for an organisation called the Children's Hours Trust. Despite the official sounding name, the work took place in the unkempt dilapidated local authority flat of an 80-year-old maverick pioneer, Rachel Pinney (Pinney et al., 1983), who did extraordinary work with autistic children. Rachel's living room was the playroom, her kitchen the staffroom and no one had police checks. These were heady innovative days, too unlicensed for today, but life-changing work was done. Rachel's level of empathy with the children was profound, children changed dramatically, but her tough training required dispensing with much that felt natural. She taught us to really stay with a child's actual immediate experience, to follow their play, reflect their actions and feeling back to them, never direct, interpret or explain, just stay true to their emotional and bodily experience.

Rachel was a tough taskmaster. We trainees paired up, did role plays, exposed our feelings and learnt how our own preoccupations and 'issues' could play havoc with the seemingly simple act of empathy. Co-counselling was the rage back then, and we gained a deep experience of being genuinely listened to and understood. This was new in my life and soon took me back into my own therapy several times a week. I felt deep relief, especially from allowing parts of me that I had hidden from myself and others to come into the light, breathe, be seen and accepted. This was where I learnt deeply of the benefits of empathy and compassion, and there has been no looking back.

In the playroom, time and again children calmed down when receiving such attuned attention. They then started to play imaginatively, working through central life issues with a fierce, intensity, often leading to symptoms abating. Yet it was easy to disrupt this flow. Their play faltered if my attention wandered, if I miscued, or my empathy was not on the button. For example, Joey, a deprived all-over-the-place 8-year-old dramatically calmed down when his play was followed and he could trust in my benign attention. Yet the moment my mind tensed, even though I retained the same external physical stance, he became dysregulated, even aggressive. As Donald Winnicott (1971) taught us long ago, being held in mind gives rise to a deep sense of ease. However, sadly, feeling held in the mind (and heart) of another is often a new and hard-to-trust experience for deprived children.

Rachel's philosophy had a profound influence on me. Early in my therapy training I was earning money working in a parent-run nursery. A little boy, who I call Ethan, was crying and shouting. The other workers were getting desperate, as we had a long walk to navigate to make the lunch we were late for. Attempts to cajole Ethan simply exacerbated his entrenched crying, protesting and shouting. One parent-worker tried to persuade him, another tried telling him off, and another to yank him along the road. It all made it worse. I decided to see if the Rachel Pinney method could help. Self-consciously I sidled up to Ethan. He looked at me and winced. I said clearly, while keeping my distance, 'Oh no, you are not sure what this other grown-up will want.' Ethan calmed a little. I said with some force, 'You are so so angry about having to go.' The tension in his jaw softened slightly. 'It's just not fair is it? He looked at me long and hard. 'I wonder what is most unfair?' His lips quivered slightly, I said aloud quietly to myself, 'Yes I wonder, I really want to know, if Ethan wants to tell me.' After what seemed an eternity he whispered, looking down and away, 'My horsey'. 'Your horsey, goodness, what happened?' 'Susan.' 'What, Susan … (I guessed) has your horsey?' He looked down. I said tentatively, 'The horsey you had?' He nodded mournfully. 'Oh how really upsetting. Shall I speak to Susan?' He nodded again, slightly glancing at me. 'Shall we do this together after lunch?' He nodded. 'Ok, perhaps you can come with me now,' I said, holding out my hand, and along he came. I had feared egg on my face and suddenly I felt like I possessed some magic. Just the act of bearing and staying with his feelings allowed him to soften and become trusting.

This was no miracle, just a basic life skill, but one that felt revelatory to me, possibly because I had received little of such attention myself. Often, I wish all trainee therapists learnt basic non-directive counselling before using more complex depth psychology thinking with children.

My perspectives

However, therapeutic alliances are about more than empathy, attunement or Carl Roger's (1957) 'unconditional positive regard'. Empathy and compassion are multi-facetted and complex and certainly not just sweetly 'nicey-nice'. They require courage and the ability to escort people into dark, uncomfortable places. Good therapeutic work also requires thorough trainings, including an in-depth knowledge of theories. Knowing how to speak to and be with another in helpful ways, while being present with ourselves, come from personal and professional experience, training, personal therapy, aptitude, being well supervised and importantly, from not being too certain, and being prepared to learn from mistakes.

In *Nurturing Natures* (Music, 2016) I used the classical metaphor of the blind man and the elephant. Here, each blind man has a definite yet limited perspective on a single part of an elephant, but each adamantly insists that their perspective is what the elephant 'really is'. To understand emotional development, we need knowledge from many disciplines, such as attachment theory, neurobiology, systemic thinking, anthropology, psychoanalysis, behavioural theory, evolutionary psychology and more. While lurching between a cocktail of eclectic influences is unlikely to help anyone, especially if it unsteadies a practitioner, we need to be open to new ideas, and integrate them into our practice, into our philosophy and, most importantly, into our very beings.

The lives of those we work with are too precious and developmental opportunities too few to waste time trying to prove what we already believe. As Einstein is reported to have said, 'it is not sane to keep doing the same things again and again yet expect different results'. We can all be guilty of repeating our favourite habits, and avoiding feeling uncertain. Worst of all is repeating old habits and, when they are not effective, blaming the recipient for being resistant!

Therapeutically my most profound influence has been, and I suspect always will be, psychoanalysis, with its emphasis on non-conscious and unconscious processes, its ability to bear the harshest of realities, its capacity to understand defensive coping mechanisms, so-called defences originally erected as adaptive strategies but that since have become maladaptive.

Psychoanalysis is my bedrock, an anchor to return to, a secure base from where I explore. From psychoanalysis, I gain deep relief in knowing that the most unbearable and unthinkable experiences can be borne and thought about. There are no shortcuts to staying with the darkest of experiences, those aspects of human nature we might prefer to disavow. Psychoanalysis teaches us how our minds play tricks, keeping us ignorant of our deepest motivations, denying realities we don't want to face.

From psychoanalysis, I learnt an ingredient missing from my somewhat naïve Rachel Pinney days, the importance of projection. The feelings stirred up in us when with disturbed children, whether anger, frustration, inadequacy, are often feelings that the child or young person has known all too well but cannot yet process. Oftentimes they are desperate to be rid of such feelings, including by 'evacuation', that is, getting another to feel them instead, rather like kicking the cat after a bad day.

Ryan, for example, often tried to denigrate and humiliate me, making me feel stupid. I often dreaded our sessions. He stated with cold venom that I was an idiot therapist, incapable of helping anyone. Some years back I might have become defensive, or worse, allowed his statements to trigger my own shame. In time, I learnt that kids like Ryan had themselves been humiliated and ridiculed and part of my role was to process in myself feelings that he knew all too well. I needed to know from the inside what he had suffered, before I could help him manage such excruciating experiences. Many stories that follow have similar examples.

Other influences on my work include attachment theory, which has provided huge understanding of troubled children and adults. Alongside it, developmental science as pioneered by the likes of Daniel Stern (1985) has greatly enriched my work, teaching us about the importance of attunement, empathy, mismatches and repairs, and intersubjective potential. Such developmental understandings provide vital lessons for therapeutic and other relationships (Boston Process of Change Group, 2010).

Alongside attachment theory, evolutionary psychology teaches how our traits, whether anxious, reactive, calm or trusting, start as adaptive responses to early environments, but can backfire later in life. As trauma therapist and neuroscientist Bruce Perry (Perry et al., 1995) stated, our early 'states' become 'traits'. In a violent home where survival depends on being distrustful, vigilant and reactive, it makes no sense to be calmly easeful. Such initial 'adaptations' can though become problems later, in school, work or relationships.

Thus, people's presentations are best understood via current and early environments. Donald Winnicott (1965) famously stated that there is no such thing as a baby, only an infant in relationship with significant others. Systemic thinking adds a vital ingredient by emphasising how we are all living in and influenced by contexts, embedded in cultures, ecological systems (Bronfenbrenner, 2004) and power relations (Foucault, 2002).

In stories that follow I describe balancing the capacity of psychoanalysis to bear the darkest in human experience with new understandings of how we help grow positive emotions, such as hope and resilience. The positive psychology movement (Goleman, 2006), mindfulness and Gilbert's (2014) compassion-focused therapy are but three of many therapeutic modalities that balance hope and pain. We meet many in these pages who have never dared embrace hope, trust, enjoyment or safeness. For those with pessimistic 'Eeyore-ish' bents, and I include myself in that group, embracing hope or pleasure can be daunting.

Eastern thought and mindfulness infuse my every session, teaching so much about attending to whatever is present in our moment-to-moment experience, rather than being aversive to it. As mindfulness suggests, it requires 'effortful effortlessness' to non-judgementally attend to both another human being and one's own feeling and body states, with interest and compassion. Mindfulness includes both a concentrated form of attention, such as on one's breath, as well as the ability to use a more open-focused form of awareness, such as on sounds or body-states generally. Attending to another human being requires similar skills, being able to hone in on states of mind, to have insights, while retaining the open, wide form of attention that psychoanalysts call 'free-floating'.

Neurobiology, while still in its infancy, has opened new vistas on body states, brains and nervous systems and how these are affected by trauma, changing how we work with maltreatment, abuse and neglect. Traumatised children are living with troubled minds and feelings, their traumas generally carried non-consciously in their bodies (van der Kolk, 2014). We are learning to work with body states as a site of intervention, to become body aware of both those we work with and ourselves. Personally I rely a lot on my own mindfulness and yoga practices, alongside supervision, to develop such capacities.

Evidence base?

Child mental health services are increasingly dominated by 'evidence-based practice' agendas and 'quick-fix' protocol-based treatments. With limited therapeutic resources, we should of course employ the best treatments, but there are downsides. Pressure from waiting lists has led to tighter top-down management, huge stress in systems (Armstrong and Rustin, 2014), and both risk-averse and fear-driven cultures. Management-driven auditing, data collection and treatment targets can be used defensively, forcing pressures onto front-line staff (Cooper and Lousada, 2005).

Being in touch with emotional pain stirs up feelings that few of us want. Institutions can defend against such discomfort with various mechanisms. People referred for treatment, who need support and under-standing, can be too quickly labelled as bearers of symptoms to which we apply a specific treatment protocol. Sometimes this helps, but often it is a way of not bearing the realities of someone's life. Isobel Menzies Lyth (1988) long ago described such a culture in hospitals where nurses referred, for example, to 'the liver in bed 12' as opposed to being present to a real, suffering human being.

Few of the children and young people populating these pages have a simple 'disorder' that can be 'treated' with a specific protocol. Many are 'co-morbid', with multiple diagnoses, such as ADHD, autistic spectrum disorders, conduct disorders and more. I suggest that what such children really need is ongoing relationships where they feel understood and can develop faith in their ability to grow, to love and be loved, to begin to heal from trauma.

Perhaps the biggest problem with the evidence-based practice agenda is that, when you drill down, the real evidence for what is effective seems to be less about the treatment modality and more about the quality of the therapeutic relationship. Many researchers have carefully examined what are called the 'common factors' (Lambert, 2005) that make for a successful outcome. The actual modality we employ, whether cognitive behavioural therapy, mentalisation, systemic family therapy, or another, often comes out as a low contributor to success. More important are human factors such as the therapeutic alliance, which is the most researched ingredient of all (Norcross and Lambert, 2014).

This does not mean that we ignore skills, therapeutic techniques or what works for whom (Fonagy *et al.*, 2005). For example, for a simple phobia, such as fear of spiders, treatments such as cognitive behavioural therapy (CBT) generally work more effectively than others. However, psychotherapy is also a craft, one in which wanting to continually learn and improve one's skills is linked with better outcomes. Research shows that some clinicians are super-therapists whose patients get better, faster, while sadly there are therapists whose patients get worse (Wampold and Wampold, 2015). Isolating the factors that make for good therapeutic work is vital, many such factors being relational, such as being curious, caring about the client, believing in the likely progress of the therapy and building a successful therapeutic alliance.

Being loyal to a specific modality, and fidelity to a treatment protocol (Norcross and Karpiak, 2017), is not a reliable predictor of good outcomes. Norcross, a major researcher in the field, argues for the importance of the human qualities of the therapist, quoting George Eliot's character Mary Ann Evans in *The Mill on the Floss* (1860) who suggested that we need people 'from a life vivid and intense enough to have created a wide fellow-feeling with all that is human' (p. 527). This echoes Wampold's and others' emphasis on the 'real relationship'. Of course it is not easy to define what is 'real' in a relationship, despite researchers developing psychotherapeutic measures of this (Gelso, 2010). However, we generally know what it is like to be on the receiving end of someone being 'genuine' as opposed to playing a role. The last thing that will help anyone is being with a caricature therapist.

The therapeutic alliance comprises a number of elements (Wampold and Wampold, 2015), perhaps most important being the bond between client and therapist and agreement about goals and tasks. Empathy, central to a successful therapeutic alliance, not surprisingly positively affects outcomes (Malin and Pos, 2015), while low empathy leads to dropouts and poor results (Moyers and Miller, 2013). This sounds obvious but is worth reiterating. Few of us want to spend intimate time revealing our deepest anxieties to someone who does not show us empathy.

Research about interpersonal bodily synchrony shows how embodied attunement, recently also termed 'embodied mentalising' (Shai and Belsky, 2017), enhances mutual trust and cooperation (LaFrance, 1979).

Feeling good comes from being in synchronous harmony with those around us. After being imitated, people tend to be more generous in subsequent encounters, and even 18-month-olds are more prosocial after being imitated (Carpenter *et al.*, 2013). Walking, singing or other acts undertaken in synchrony with others all increase cooperativeness and helpfulness (Wiltermuth and Heath, 2009). Humans are primed to join with others, to co-operate, and like many mammals, we co-regulate each other, good relationships greatly enhancing psychological and physical health.

I have noticed in sessions how the extent of mutual synchrony is enormously telling. With one person, Jade, I often realise that her body posture mirrors mine, perhaps the way her hand is on her chin, or how her legs are crossed or the angle of her head. Often, I have no idea who is leading or following, or even if it makes sense to ask that question. This happens less when relationships are more awkward.

Yet many from traumatised backgrounds struggle with interpersonal attunement, reciprocity and indeed, relationships generally. They have often missed out on the building blocks of cooperation or mutual care, lacking the capacity to receive care from even benign others. Max, adopted from a violent and neglectful home, had few friends, was rarely invited to parties or play dates and often got into conflict. With him I often found myself tense retreating from him. Our postures were dissonant, not matched, although they became more synchronous as he came to trust me more. Our embodied responses nearly always have meaning, containing vital clues, whether irritation, boredom, liking. Later I describe how our embodied countertransference responses, what gets stirred up in us in interpersonal meetings, might be as important a 'royal road to the unconscious' as Freud considered dreams to be.

One fascinating study looked at interviews with patients who had attempted suicide (Heller and Haynal, 1997). The psychiatrists' notes did not predict future suicide attempts, but what did, amazingly, were the gestures and body postures of not only the patients, but fascinatingly, also the psychiatrists in the initial video-taped interviews. With those who would re-attempt suicide over the next year, the psychiatrists were more distant, gaze aversive and frowned more. The psychiatrists would have been barely if at all conscious of such gestures, but their embodied responses were the biggest clues to the patients' states of mind.

This it is not surprising. Psychotherapy research suggests that high synchrony between therapist and patient is linked with a more positive therapeutic alliance (Koole and Tschacher, 2016). Interpersonal co-regulatory skills are generally honed very early in life, but can also be built upon in training and supervision. Without them therapeutic work is far less effective.

In fact, psychotherapy research suggests better outcomes not from perfect synchrony but when the therapist can repair interactions that have gone wrong (Safran *et al.*, 2009). Repairing of mismatches is also central to secure and attuned parent–child relationships (Beebe *et al.*, 2005). A child does not benefit from perfect interactions, nor a client from a perfectly attuned therapist. When an interaction goes awry, but the responsible adult can read the signals, and help repair it, then emotional growth and resilience results. In a therapy session, this can require honesty, authenticity and courage.

The success of a therapy is profoundly linked to the quality of the relationship. Not surprisingly, having a secure attachment to one's therapist predicts good outcomes (Lilliengren *et al.*, 2015). Attachment theory is at the heart of mentalisation approaches to psychotherapy, with its central concept of epistemic trust (Fonagy and Allison, 2014), a trust in adults such as teachers, therapists or parents who help make sense of the world. This happens mainly through the kinds of personal qualities I emphasise in this book, such as integrity, empathy, attunement, sensitivity, authenticity and the ability to be curious and compassionately in touch with our own and others' states.

The chapters

The chapters ahead are populated by therapy stories from my practice over the years. The next chapter gives granularity to concepts I describe in this introduction, such as the role of attunement, empathy and reciprocity. We hear about two cases, Josie, and a young, somewhat autistic girl, Molly, and my struggles to make emotional contact with them and allow the emergence and expression of feelings, whether rage and aggression, or hope and joy. These themes, and that of ruptures and repairs, are taken forward in Chapter 3 where Molly reappears alongside some older children, and we witness extraordinary psychological shifts including increased resilience, agency and newfound belief in life's riches.

The next chapters describe contrasting presentations through the lens of attachment theory. First, I look at what we nowadays call hyperactivated attachment styles, where people are insecure, anxious and easily triggered into threat states. For example, we meet a girl I call Grace, whose life in a chaotic family gave rise to clingy behaviour, Damian, whose history of violence led to him being easily upset and hard to soothe, and in Chapter 5, Stuart, who needed to build the capacity to self-regulate, and then develop a mind that could think thoughts.

Chapters 6 and 7 describe quite different presentations, children who are flatter, dampened down, with what we call 'deactivated' presentations. We meet Martin, a much-ignored child, who could be flat and dull, and Jenny, whose parents placed little value on emotions and had no time for neediness or upset. Jenny survived by using her mind to avoid her feelings and body states. Here I tease out the fundamental differences between the presence of bad experiences, such as trauma or violence, from the lack of good experiences, as seen in emotional neglect, each giving rise to completely different ways of making sense of and adapting to the interpersonal world.

From here I think more about trauma and the body, how we need to be aware of body states – our own and that of others. In trauma, people can become dissociated and out of touch with their own bodily signals. In Chapter 8, I describe young people like Paula who would place herself in difficult situations, in part because she could not read signals her body was sending her, such as anxiety, danger or even pleasure. She had learnt in an abusive childhood to not feel what her body might be communicating, leading to a life with too little emotional awareness.

In Chapter 9, I describe mistakes made earlier in my career when I believed my job was always to help bear pain and suffering. I eventually learnt that focusing on traumatic incidents too quickly could be profoundly unhelpful, re-triggering dissociation and flashbacks. Recent trauma theory teaches the importance of facilitating a sense of safety before processing traumas. The cases here show how easy it is to get this wrong, but also how genuine change takes place when we get it right.

The next chapters look at the best and worst of human nature. In Chapter 10 we witness how aggression take root in the personality, both a hot-blooded reactive type as well as a colder, more callous, even psychopathic type. We meet traumatised young people who move from believing that aggression and power are the only sensible ways to survive, to courageously daring to trust that goodness, trust and vulnerability are manageable and even a good idea.

In Chapter 11, we see how altruism, cooperation and kind-heartedness can get turned off by stress and trauma, but how the innate propensity to be helpful and generous can be turned back on with good-enough experiences. We meet Terry, who was in thrall to sadistic aggression, and Sophie, who replicated her cruel early life experience by attacking and hurting others. We see how, as they began to trust in me and the therapy, they softened and became kinder, and nicer to be with. They, along with Fred, whose hatred of life was directed more towards himself, all experienced a major shift towards both compassion for themselves and others.

Similar themes are seen in Chapter 12, which focuses on addictive states of mind. I look at the effects of digital technology, such as pornography or girls' risky use of social media. We examine how the modern world poses challenges that were not present when many of us were learning our trade. People who are addicted, whether to substances, gambling, pornography or other technology, in effect have bodies taken over by forces that seem to control them, while self-reflective and self-regulatory capacities get turned down. Many turn to their addiction of choice at times of stress or upset, as a way of not feeling feelings. For example, I describe Mano, who was masturbating up to 18 times a day to pornography, an addiction that took over his life. Thankfully recovery is possible, if people are helped both to bear emotional pain and regain hope in the goodness that life can offer.

The final chapter looks beyond individual development. I show how complex interpersonal dynamics can be re-enacted in professional networks and how looking beyond a child's 'behaviour' to what is going on beneath the surface is crucial. I describe a school where under pressure staff responded by becoming increasingly punitive, to manage their own understandable stresses. We see how children can become scapegoated when systems are not working well, and how reflecting upon and bearing feelings rather than acting precipitately can give rise to emotional relief, containment and a softening of attitudes. This leads to a change from seeing a child as 'bad' to perhaps seeing them as sad or unhappy. Finally, in my conclusion I offer personal reflections on the qualities needed to do this work well.

A consistent finding from psychotherapy research is that effective therapists allow themselves to be uncertain and curious, to bear not knowing, to remain open to learning (Wampold and Wampold, 2015). This would have heartened the psychoanalyst Wilfred Bion (2013) who embraced what Keats (1899) described as 'negative capability', when we are 'capable of being in uncertainties, mysteries, doubts without any irritable reaching after fact and reason' (p. 277). Being uncertain though is easier said than done. It requires trust in the unknown, a belief that if we open to novelty and put aside our cherished shibboleths, something new, meaningful and rewarding will come into that space.

This is what we see in securely attached children who, when safe, feel free to explore and be easefully curious. They know in their bones that if something untoward were to happen, an attachment figure would be there to mop things up, proffer understanding and be with them until they feel safe enough to renew exploring. Mindfulness practitioners similarly know that to be present, curious and 'awake' to the present moment requires a sense of ease and trust. This is not a flaccid, slothful relaxation, but a presence that feels alive, alert, genuinely open to experience, but not too effortful. This is the state of mind psychoanalysts describe as free-floating attention, in which we allow our minds to associate to what is happening in 'effortless effort-fullness'. I suspect that this state of mind is also the bedrock of a rich and fulfilled life, lives we hope for in those we work with.

Our work is always about reaching out respectfully to the world of the other, trying to make sense of their unique experience, values, feelings and thoughts. This means eschewing omniscience, while still learning to trust what we feel and think. Therapy, like all good relationships, is a journey, a kind of road trip, taking both parties to unexpected places, nearly always in ways that challenge both therapist and client. In meeting people in the depths of their beings, we can facilitate movement towards a life based in hope, freedom and compassion, and grow a trust that difficulty can be faced and can lead to growth. When we manage this, we often see genuine, heart-warming, exciting and profound change.

Chapter 2

One foot in the ditch

Josie: a therapeutic vignette

Josie was a 13-year-old only child who struggled with friendships. She was wary of adults, which was not surprising given the brittleness and busyness of her high-flying businesswoman mother and academic father, neither of whom had enough time for her. She was in therapy due to anxiety and depressive symptoms. About six months into therapy she entered my room, smiled, looked around and I noticed her smile shift into a momentary grimace. I sensed that her evident disapproval was meaningful but I ignored my feeling.

This was a mistake; such fleeting feeling states nearly always have meaning. She began fidgeting, her body posture tense, distant, barely meeting my eyes. I asked if she was cross or upset. She brushed me aside irritably. I wondered if there was something from the last session that was riling her, or had something happened at school or at home? No response. I felt incompetent, but also noted my frustration, feeling that I was being punished. This went on for some time.

She determinedly resisted me for a while, but eventually softened slightly, and I caught a darting look towards the edge of the room, near the couch. Sticking out, just visible, was a young girl's glove.

Last week I had given her my next holiday dates. She had seemed somewhat frosty. The glove though was a blatant reminder of my other life. She assumed I had children who claimed most of my attention. She also had begun to realise that I see other patients, a fact that she, like many, had mostly been able to keep out of her mind. The sight of the glove felt like being hit with a wet flannel of reality. This all crystallised in that fleeting moment when her eyes darted across the room, and my heart dipped. My earlier bodily reaction was a clue I wrongly ignored.

I had a choice now. I had been contemptuously brushed aside so often that I was tempted to shirk another fight. Yet I knew Josie's central issue was being gifted to me in the session, which was her belief that those she needed did not have enough time or mental space for her, an issue alive here and now with me.

I had to phrase anything I said carefully. Even saying 'You are upset that . . .' might trigger a defensive rebuttal, as if I was humiliating her, showing condescending pity. Josie had a lifetime's defences against feeling needy and vulnerable, and had worked hard to avoid emotional pain, which she found intolerable, prompting retreat at the slightest hint of rejection.

Taking a deep breath, I said, 'Oh goodness, it was so thoughtless to leave that glove lying around.' I waited, noting a slight unstiffening and simultaneous pursing. I risked carrying on, saying in a slightly theatrical, but still serious way, 'If I was paying proper attention to anyone coming here, I would protect them more carefully from other parts of my life.' I was careful to avoid any hint that she was more vulnerable than anyone else, so I kept it general rather than address her particular upset. She was not ready to face her distress until she was in touch with her first line of defence, anger at being let down. As I allowed myself to be the object of her anger, her relief was palpable. She knew that I knew that she was upset, that feelings of rejection had been triggered. But she needed to experience anger and disappointment first, and I needed to be strong enough to take it. I said, 'This could just prove that I am not a reliable or trustworthy enough person for you.' Her breathing deepened slightly.

Admitting feeling hurt was still too much. I said, 'And it is not as if this is the first time that people have been thoughtless about your feelings.' While this might be seen as me evading her angry feelings, it in fact allowed her to come to them at her own pace, with trust that I was not going to rub her nose in her vulnerability. I was, as Meltzer (2008) described, 'tip-toeing up to pain'. She could then talk about her parents having no time for her. This was an old story. What was new was letting painful feelings through, real sadness about what she did not receive but so yearned for, perhaps for the first time allowing feelings of longing and loss.

I asked what she would have wanted that she did not get. Josie tearfully described how she had felt humiliated for having needs. For the first time, she could safely re-experience these feelings in my presence, as if they were, as she would later say, safely blanketed in my thought and care. These remained hard feelings to bear, she still hated them, but there was now hope that such feelings could be borne, not just disavowed.

Of course, this was the beginning not the end of a journey. Josie had organised much of her personality around avoiding feelings that as a young child were unbearable. Yet refusing to feel such feelings was now increasingly causing her problems.

As always, such issues needed delicate handling. The clues were in the emotionally alive experience in the room with me, the transference, as manifested in the glove, her fleeting expression, my body tightening. In time, I would need to help her process not only anger, but also her neediness, yearning and fear of rejection. These cannot be fudged, but nor can they be rushed. Eventually she would learn that the vulnerable needy feelings she was so terrified of, which led to humiliation in her childhood, might become bearable.

The great paediatrician, Donald Winnicott (1953), once wrote that the fear of breakdown is generally the fear of something that in fact had happened long ago, often in infancy, He was purported to have said, 'Tell me what you fear and I will tell you what happened to you'. In other words, we expend huge amounts of energy forcing stable doors closed long after the horse has bolted, bracing in the present against past threats. Therapy holds out the hope that the experiences we expend so much psychic effort avoiding might not any longer be as bad as we fear.

This means exploring such feelings, investigating their bodily expression, surfing the waves of their sensations, befriending and taming them. If this works, then so much time and energy need no longer be spent building fortresses to avoid painful emotional states. In fact, such fortresses often take us out of life more than the original experiences did. Josie needed me to struggle to be with her, to tentatively offer compassionate care, so she might in time give such compassion to herself.

Empathy, therapeutic alliances and compassionate companions

Possibly the best therapy lesson I ever received was from a now deceased but brilliant teacher at the Minster Centre, Dennis Hyde, when I started training. We were role playing being clients and therapists. Most of us were either overly empathic or distant. Dennis suggested that when you are in emotional trouble, it is like being stuck in a ditch. You want someone to reach down to you in the ditch. But if we get too far into the ditch and can't get out either, we are no help. Then there are two people stuck in the dark hole. Equally if we are too high above the ditch, waving, we seem too distant and aloof. We need to keep one of our feet firmly in the ditch and the other on the bank, and reach in with a firm hand and a belief that they can be pulled out. This has stayed with me as brilliant advice. In fact, people's ditches come in many shapes and depths, and how we position ourselves in relation to each person's ditch will be different. Much good therapeutic work is in working out how to angle our bodies, direct our eyes, pitch our voices and frame our sentences in order to most helpfully reach the other.

Dennis was really talking about empathy, that ability to not just know someone else's feelings, but to feel with them. Empathy comes from a German word *einfühlung*, meaning 'feeling into'. It suggests cultivating a place in ourselves where another's emotions can be processed. Wilfred Bion (1962b) called this containment, using the metaphor of the stomach digesting and metabolising an experience, in effect detoxifying it. A good parent or therapist, having processed a child's experience, can find a way to present back an understanding of that experience in safely metabolised form.

As in Josie's case, this is easier said than done. I learnt tough lessons, of getting too close to Josie in her ditch, and her recoiling with anger, or being too distant, and her feeling that I was aloof. The exact angle at which I placed myself was crucial. For example, she could not initially allow me to feel 'for her'. In talking to her hurt self, I beamed a spotlight on to a part of her that she was not yet ready to acknowledge. She could experience my genuine empathy as patronising. In the example above, when she was upset, I did not use the word 'you', but rather talked about my mistake and how annoying that must be. This was angling my position in what is called a 'therapist-centered' (Steiner, 1994) way, so that she could take in my understanding without feeling threatened.

Compassion is too soft or 'heart-based' a word for some, but in effective therapy I have no doubt that compassion and caring about the other's plight is central. Acknowledging this, but not in a desperate way, can have a profound effect. If we are overwhelmed by another's feelings, we can overreact, and possibly clients will experience their own feelings boomeranging back unprocessed from our own struggling psyche. Similarly, attempts to help by offering brilliant strategies can feel like we cannot bear their feelings or plight. Yet not showing our care for another's suffering will be experienced as cold and distant, waving from far above that ditch.

I now take forward such thinking with an extended example.

Molly

My first glimpse of 4-year-old Molly was of a spindly, slight, blond waif, somewhat wild-eyed, in her own world. She was the third and final child, referred because of constant emotional meltdowns. Molly's mother described her as 'difficult from birth', hard to soothe and having 'cried and cried'. Molly from the get-go was hypersensitive to external stimuli, with a tendency to easily feel overwhelmed, and then withdraw.

I was lucky to see her in twice-weekly therapy. She could bear little frustration, hated change and easily fell into despairing states. This was a major challenge for a newish therapist wanting to empathise. My temptation was to show how I could stay with her despair, which for many children would have helped. For Molly, this felt like I was too much inside the ditch with her. Seeing her pain reflected in my face made her feel that there was no escaping her despair.

Although Molly was a planned and wanted child, the period around her birth was stressful due to family crises. Her parents struggled with emotional attunement anyway, and at Molly's birth were less available than usual. They had experienced few problems with their older children, born at less stressful times and possibly Molly was constitutionally less robust. Molly's sensitivity alongside the unusual family-life stressors may have led to her specific difficulties.

Whatever the aetiology, her prognosis was looking bad. Her despairing moods smacked already of depression. Worryingly, many of her behaviours suggested a child moving on to the autistic spectrum. For example, she could do a 300-piece jigsaw with the pieces turned upside down, yet would cling rigidly to routines, unable to bear change or spontaneity. She did not play imaginatively, had never babbled as a baby, her speech was delayed, comprehension minimal. She did not feel the cold, as if living in an ethereal disembodied state, and spent a lot of time withdrawn, engaging in repetitive activities. I felt I was in the presence of a delicate flower with whom I had to be terribly careful.

In early sessions, she lined up toy animals, while I failed to realise that her almost undetectable mouth movements were naming the animals to herself, seemingly unaware of my presence. She lacked any idea of another who could be with her, hear her, who she might have an impact on. The muffled sounds from under her breath were probably attempts at what researchers call proto-conversations (Bateson, 1971), early attempts by babies to communicate. She did not lift her head as she 'spoke' and it was hard to believe that these emotionless dulled sounds were directed at me or anyone. I imagine that she was ungratifying to parent as she gave out little of what evokes positive responses in parents.

She gave up on things easily and was plunged into despair by the slightest setback. Trying to put two pieces of toy fencing together she said despairingly, 'I can't,' and wailed, 'I wanna see mummy.' The psychotherapist Francis Tustin (1992), who had extraordinary insights into autistic children, noted that 'such a child expects to do everything at the first attempt ... when he fails he desists from effort' (p. 111). This fitted Molly only too well. She became fearful on hearing slight noises that I barely registered, giving up on activities in desultory fashion at the first hurdle. She flitted from activity to activity, seemingly blown by whatever sensation overtook her in the moment. When she saw me in the waiting room she always passively sat still until I called her. I had to be extremely attuned to her emotional states or else she would retreat. I knew I had to show her that there was life outside the ditch.

Empathy is not enough

Early sessions often consisted of trying to stay attuned to her emotional states. I would 'mark' (Fonagy *et al.*, 2004) her emotions, making simple sounds that caught or slightly exaggerated her feeling tone, to show that I understood, took seriously but was not overwhelmed by her experience (one foot in and one out of the ditch). I spent time just naming feelings, saying things like, 'That's hard, you couldn't do it', or 'Oh dear, that makes you very sad', conveying a sense that her feelings could be borne and processed.

For a long time, this made little difference and, like her, I nearly lost heart. In one session, some months into the work, after her mother left she again became very upset. I responded by trying to show that I understood her, making comments with feeling like, 'Oh dear, how upset Molly is, you're missing your mummy.' When I added, 'So annoying, it is just not fair', she began to look at me with interest. She was calmed by feeling understood, but especially by my suggestion that protest was possible, that outside the ditch of despair there was another potential perspective, other feeling states.

This is perhaps straightforward, what most thoughtful workers or parents do, showing how feelings can be borne and processed. When I said something like, 'That is so upsetting', my voice carried tones of sadness but also some force. In response, Molly looked at me long and hard and relaxed, knowing that I understood her feelings from the inside, but was also processing them from outside the ditch. I was helping Molly to recognise her own states of mind in a safe, 'marked' (Fonagy *et al.*, 2004), metabolised (Bion, 1962b) form. She was experiencing what Winnicott (1971) described when he stated, 'What does the infant see when he looks at his mother? He sees himself' (p. 131), and a belief that her feelings were manageable was taking root.

Too often I empathised with her sadness, which only led her to get sadder, as if her nose was being rubbed in despair she was already too familiar with. I also needed to be in touch with her potential strength and outrage, to enable her to trust in her agency and power, not just face difficult feelings. Being sad for some can be an achievement, while for others like Molly it is too linked with given-up states, a form of learned helplessness (Peterson *et al.*, 1993).

Things shifted when I learnt to amplify hints of stronger feelings, like anger or passion. When in one session she threw a toy giraffe on the floor I exaggerated her feeling, saying, 'You really want to throw that silly giraffe away.' She smiled and jumped on the table, swinging the giraffe with almost a hint of triumph.

Here is a classic therapeutic dilemma. Often a therapist's natural response is to be empathic to a victim, such as the 'poor giraffe', all tied up and forgotten about. Indeed, we might often hear a parent or worker say something like, 'You are not being very nice to the poor giraffe.' However, Molly needed others to help her bear her strength and anger, and drawing attention to the 'poor' giraffe led to a loss of energy, re-triggering fears and anxieties. On the other hand, she came alive when her strength and vitality were echoed and encouraged.

Reciprocity

For months, there was little reciprocal play. Then in one session, as she picked up some string, something in her body language allowed me to say, 'You've got the string', in a way that showed that I expected a response. She said, 'Dring', mirroring me, but for once not in a flat compliant way, and I said, holding my breath, 'Yes, string'. This does not sound like much but in fact was real progress. My presence and attention had helped allow her to communicate, even be playful, almost the first sign of reciprocal interaction.

More elaborate playing soon followed. She took the toy tea set, signalling that we both drink pretend tea. I spontaneously said 'cheers' and Molly laughed, imitating my tone, taking on my enjoyment and enthusiasm. Shared songs followed in the forthcoming months, games like pat-a-cake and London Bridge is falling down. Molly was finding reciprocity less dangerous than she had feared. Trust was developing that someone could be 'in sync' with her and not overwhelm her. Her autistic features started to recede.

This new-found faith in interpersonal interactions contrasted with her early presentation. In our initial assessment Molly had drawn her a primitive picture of a person. I was silently thrilled. Her mother asked, 'Who is the picture of?' and when Molly quietly muttered, 'Daddy' she was brusquely asked, 'Where is his beard?' Molly's face fell, liveliness melted away, the paper and crayons discarded and not returned to for months. Molly's mother unwittingly and with good intentions, had 'broken up' a tentative exploratory gesture. Molly would jump if anyone coughed, startle at a noise 200 yards away, and withdrew at a slightly raised voice. That excruciating moment was possibly all too typical of a misfit between a temperamentally sensitive child and a somewhat preoccupied parent.

Molly's mother's communications were often experienced as a harsh, even jagged, otherness, rather than a softer, attuned one. Molly fitted well the description brilliantly penned by Anne Alvarez (1992), of being 'undrawn', rather than withdrawn. Her hypersensitivity could lead her to quickly retreat, or appear lifeless, even depressed.

I learnt, when she showed even slight upset, to speak not to the despair but to the potent or angry parts of her. I often rhythmically banged out the emotional tone of my words on a table. Initially she looked at me in surprise. In one session she noticed that the doll's house beds were not where she had last left them. She began sorting them with a hint of displeasure. I exaggerated this, saying. 'You are very upset and angry, Mr Music put that bed in the wrong place', and, 'Molly wants the beds upstairs not downstairs, she is putting them just where *she* wants them', emphasising the 'she'. To my surprise she banged the table in feeling response to my words. My colleagues at the Tavistock, Peter Hobson and Tony Lee (1989), described how autistic children struggle to identify with others, mimicking surface appearances but unable to resonate with the inner bodily emotional feeling of others. This was becoming less true of Molly.

This was no longer empty mimicking, but something genuinely alive. She picked up a toy phone, looked briefly at me, and said, 'Hello Mr Mugi'. I took another, saying, 'Hello Molly, how are you?' She mumbled something, the words not quite coming, quickly putting the phone down. In forthcoming weeks such interactions became longer, characterised by increased mutuality. Molly's interactions were still barely verbal, but as research shows (Trevarthen, 2016), such gestural and rhythmic interaction are the precursors of language. Genuinely alive play was now occurring and real feelings were present. She was gaining trust in the alive presence of others, including myself and also a part of herself, an internal object, as we say in psychoanalysis, that could really listen to her.

Good aggression, libido and life

Molly's parents unfortunately were so worried about cognitive delay that they pushed her to conform to developmental milestones, such as naming colours and forming letters. She often went along with this, even basking in their praise, but what other more robust children might have experienced as helpful, Molly felt as intrusive demands, leading to compliance.

To start with my very presence often also seemed intrusive. I had to speak slowly and softly, being careful about physical proximity. She would frequently suggest 'you go there', or ask me to hide and then not come to find me. I eventually realised that she was regulating the distance between us. I often had to wait silently, knowing that any movement, let alone move towards her, would disturb her fragile equilibrium. Often for as long as 20 excruciating minutes, I remained still and quiet, awkward in my inactivity, thinking that I could not possibly justify my NHS salary in doing so little, worrying that I had been entirely forgotten about. However, in time she always re-emerged, proud of something she had made all by herself. She needed me to be sufficiently apart from her, but still present, so that she could both forget about me, yet trust I was there. Worrying less about an intrusive other, she could get on with just 'being', experiencing what Winnicott (1953) described as 'being alone in the presence of another'.

Initially, Molly was like the infants that Beebe and Lachmann (2002) described, whose insecure attachment styles meant they could only maintain eye contact with their mothers if they increased self-comforting behaviours, such as rubbing their bodies or clasping their hands. Beebe described the angle of their heads as 'cocked for escape'. Secure infants, on the other hand, look at their mothers full in the face, expecting good experiences of joining and separating. Molly needed space to feel separate, to not worry about the other, but she also needed to know I was there when needed. Through such experiences she began to become her own person.

Being with but outside despair

We learn the crucial skill of knowing our own thoughts and feelings via our mental states being 'marked' and understood by 'mind-minded' others

(Meins *et al.*, 2002), and this is fundamentally linked to securely attachment. This slowly happened for Molly, albeit not without plenty of challenges.

She often rushed from activity to activity, with no room for stillness. She lacked what Klein (1975) would call a good internal object and the experience that Winnicott (1965) described as 'going on being'. She often tried to force me into joining her frenetic activities, which I acceded to initially to avoid her pits of despair. Slowly though, I saw signs that she could manage more frustration and to her dismay I began to refuse to join in. I felt cruel, but was sure by now that she could manage some disappointment, and that this could be a growth point.

She would scream 'Come on Mr Mugi, NOW!' in fury. I took courage and momentarily stepped outside the activity, saying things like, 'I am thinking'. Molly hated this at first. This was reminiscent of the psychoanalyst, Ron Britton's (Britton et al., 1989) example of a patient who felt abandoned when Britton was clearly reflecting. Britton's patient even screamed, 'Stop that fucking thinking!' In time Molly began to tolerate and even get interested in me as a thinker, becoming more able to pause from the ceaseless activity that had previously held her together. When, rarely, she would hesitate between activities I would seize the moment and say things like, 'Molly is wondering what to do ... now what will it be? Uuumm ... I wonder ...', comments that she soon began to mimic and eventually became stepping stones for her nascent cognitive development. Soon her play became punctuated with statements like 'Now I gonna do ... let me see ... um ... I think I gonna ...'. She could now think a bit, self-observe, even use language and think playfully.

The space that developed in her mind, and between us, allowed us to be more separate, giving her breathing space. My breathing literally deepened when she felt more contained and I think hers did too. She was becoming more able to see me as separate, was less hypervigilant, less wary, more able to look at me, as if discovering my subjectivity (Benjamin, 1998).

In one session, while playing, she said, 'I scratch my head', an ordinary comment for most children, but in her a new sign of 'self-awareness'. The 'I scratch my head' was a communication from one part of herself to another, a form of self-observation. I simply replied, 'Yes, you have really noticed that you want to scratch your head.' At the end of this session she suddenly picked up a perspex ruler, which became a camera as she said, 'Say sausages' and pretended to take my picture. Like with the camera, there was a space in her mind now from which to picture her newly developing sense of self.

As I became less dangerous, she became curious about me and my mind, drawing my attention to things and looking for my reactions. This was a move towards what Trevarthen and Hubley (1978) called 'secondary intersubjectivity', two people knowing and appreciating what is in the other's mind, something that normally develops towards the end of the first year.

She would run into the therapy room before me and hide, letting me be the one experiencing the waiting. In one session, she even placed a blanket on the floor just where she sometimes hid, and placed a pillow under it, and then she hid elsewhere. This showed that she was developing a real understanding of other minds, predicting my reaction to her pretend hiding place.

Molly's mother was also getting help and becoming happier and less intrusive. She started to understand how Molly was different from her other kids. Flexibility was developing in both Molly and her mother, more ability to 'go with the flow', even more playfulness. This tends to come alongside a growing sense of security.

In one session, she heard a siren outside that I had not even noticed, something that might once have led to a dissociated freezing. She asked, 'What that noise?' I repeated the question and she said, 'It a bit like a police car.' I repeated 'a bit like the police car', marvelling at and emphasising the 'a bit like', which hinted at a mind at work. She said, 'Yes it like a police, maybe it chase some robber.' I said, 'Oh the police maybe are chasing a robber', excited at this evidence of fantasy. She said, 'Yes the robber come to my house and stole lipstick and I ran after fast.' This was a truly exciting moment. A while back she would have reacted to such a noise as a literal danger, but this noise was now being integrated into her play so it could be worked with symbolically. Molly, who we meet again in the next chapter, was now on the move, able to symbolise, be playful, gaining a capacity for both closeness and separateness, able to notice states of mind in herself and others, able to have a foot both in and out of her own ditch.

Chapter 3

Resilience, mismatches and repair

Finding potency: Michael

Michael was 17 years old, unconfident, inhibited, with few friends, was sometimes bullied and often felt judged by others. He would become infatuated with girls who were put off by the neediness he exuded. He was insightful, aware of his feelings but stuck in self-defeating patterns. His father had been cruel, teasing and had suddenly died when Michael was 7 years old. He was the youngest sibling, relying hugely on his mother who alternated between closeness and withdrawal.

For his first year of therapy, managing his huge despair seemed all that was possible. Several rejections by girls fuelled desperation and self-hating thinking. The empathy I offered at first gave relief but soon seemed unhelpful. I found myself wanting to give him a push, a 'kick up the backside', but feared this was re-enacting how he himself and others despised his 'little boy' ways.

If I 'acted in', such as when my disappointment in his inertia leaked out, he withdrew, passive-aggressively. When I stayed with how upset he was with me, he gained hope that it might be ok to disagree with me, even safe to challenge me, and his mood shifted.

In one session, I mentioned the impending break. He clearly wanted to talk about other things. I belatedly said, 'It looks like I have imposed my agenda on the session.' 'Oh no,' he said, 'you are right, thank you.' I did not accept his false compliance, suggesting not only that I might have made a mistake, but that he had a right to be fed up about this. Some colour and energy came into his cheeks.

In another session, I was a full minute late opening the door, leaving him uncertain about whether I was even there. He smiled as politely as ever, and we got on with the session. When material crept into the session about him being kept waiting by a friend, and how unpunctual his mother was, the penny dropped! I talked firmly about how unsettling it was to be kept waiting by me, how badly treated he must feel. 'Oh no, not at all', he said, but by now we knew each other well. 'Oh no,' I mimicked, 'come on! What did you want to say to your friend?' He was able to state that he disliked being treated like that. Then, to my amazement, he said, 'I deserve more respect than that!' 'Yes,' I exclaimed, 'including from me.' Energy came into his face, more muscle tone appeared. I saw a potentially strong young man and actually felt proudly paternal.

He had another rebuff from a girl, one who I thought he had a chance with, and described an unconvincing excuse she gave for cancelling a meeting. He plaintively describing his fear that he would never have a relationship, 'martyrishly' complaining that girls do not want nice guys, that 'bastards' always win. His anger gave me heart, and as he looked up forlornly I surprised myself by saying, 'Aren't you going to fight for her?' Equally surprisingly he did, and with some success. He slowly, with the support of therapy, and a new male friend, began to take more risks and act assertively, with this girl, but also with teachers, his mother and, alas, me too!

Michael still found life tough, at times excruciating, but stronger personality traits were growing, and with it a belief that setbacks needn't be disasters. Even when this relationship ended his despair had a different quality. He was angry, upset, yet less self-hating. He genuinely felt something good might be around the corner, even taking positives from the experience. Like Molly, he no longer just sunk into a default pit of despair. Sometimes I would still sympathise with his despair but often I could challenge him to rise above the belief that all would forever be doom and gloom. Then he often smiled, re-finding optimism, no longer a passive victim.

A growing part of Michael was now on the side of what the inspirational psychoanalyst Neville Symington (1993) called the 'life-giver', a part of the self that does not turn away from life or refuse hope. Symington, a psychoanalyst who does not shrink from the dark side, nonetheless maintained a central place for hope. He wrote 'turning away from the life-giver is a turning against the self. Life is potential for growth' (p. 41). There are tricky tightropes between empathising with pain, but not indulging in masochistic hopelessness, between being kind to our fear but not giving in to it, between daring to face despair and risking being powerful. It is from siding with the 'life-giver' that we grow and flourish.

Michael was developing confidence that he could take charge of his destiny. Having some control of one's situation reduces stress and aids psychological health and resilience. In 'learned helplessness' (Peterson *et al.*, 1993), animals are given major stressors, such as electric shocks. Some have some control, such as a lever that could stop the shocks, and those with such control became less hopeless, while those without the lever become despairing and fearful, exhibiting symptoms rather like human depression. Similarly, babies whose parents are unpredictable, abusive or unresponsive become more stressed and less confident than those whose wishes and feelings are responded to. If we believe we cannot affect our predicament, we stop seeing possibilities that in fact might be right in front of us.

Ruptures and repairs: Samantha and Jimmy

Samantha was 7 years old and had been with foster carers for nine months. Her mother had a history of violent relationships and Samantha had witnessed, and probably experienced, toxic amounts of violence. She was anxious, vigilant and often paralysed by fear. She was intelligent, according to psychological tests, but struggled to concentrate and did badly academically. Witnessing domestic violence has powerful effects on brains and nervous systems (McTavish *et al.*, 2016), often worse effects than being the recipient of violence oneself (Teicher and Samson, 2016).

Prior to starting a psychotherapy assessment, I organised a trainee to observe Samantha in school. We saw several examples of her frozenness. In playtime, she was invited to join in a typical if slightly complex skipping game. She tried a few steps, made a small mistake and withdrew, wearing a look of profound shame. She did not try again. In the class-room, she was desperate to please her teacher but was excruciatingly fearful of making mistakes. When asked a question she froze, even if she knew the answer. In her psychic world, and family of origin, getting something wrong, being disappointing to another, could signal impending terror and humiliation. When Samantha had started school, it was not uncommon for her to lose bladder control, presumably in panic, when feeling under pressure.

In her psychotherapy assessment, I had to be extremely cautious, especially being a man. I felt uncomfortably powerful, as if I could blow her over. In sessions she dared not explore, use toys, play or speak unless spoken to. She retreated to safe activities, stereotypical pictures of nice doll-like girls or houses with pretty gardens. Her truer feelings and grimmer inner world leaked out unconsciously in pictures, a red mark on a dress that looked like blood, ominously scary clouds above the house, trees barely rooted that could easily blow over. After the assessment, she transferred to a female therapist. Her poor confidence and predisposition to freeze was having a really bad effect on her life. Luckily this was just what could be worked with in therapy, and with her thoughtful foster carers.

Samantha had little belief that bad situations could be recovered from. Yet it is exactly such a belief that mismatches and ruptures could be recovered from that bodes well for emotional health and is seen in successful psychotherapy (Safran *et al.*, 2009).

This is partly why the classic 'still-face' procedure, developed by Tronick (2007), is so revealing. Here, a mother is asked to interact ordinarily with her infant, and then signalled to hold an expressionless face for up to two minutes. Infants generally are perplexed and disturbed, feeling 'this is not what is meant to happen'. Some work hard to re-initiate interaction, others display negative expressions such as grimacing and others manage by looking away, cutting off or self-soothing.

If they have had good-enough early experiences, infants generally try actively to get the mother to re-engage, perhaps by pointing, smiling or gesturing. Some though quickly give up, turning hopelessly inwards, in what the pioneer of infant observation, Esther Bick (1968), called 'second skin defences'. This is when we see gaze aversion, self-soothing and little belief that acting on the world, or interacting with another, can remedy a situation.

Possibly Samantha might have become frozen in a still-face experiment, assuming her mother's expressionless face presaged danger. Other passive babies, perhaps like Michael, might not freeze but lack the confidence to repair the interaction in the way secure children might.

When a mother comes out of a still face, insecure infants recover less quickly, their stress levels remaining higher than confident secure children. If a baby's signals are habitually ignored, then momentary coping mechanisms turn into ongoing patterns, leading to giving up on even kindly empathic adults.

Some children recover better from knocks, or even traumas. Jimmy, a much-loved child, was just 9 years old when his father died in a freak climbing accident. His mother fell apart and Jimmy became flat, given-up, in effect his world was falling apart. Yet Jimmy, and his mother, could use therapy to go through classic mourning symptoms, such as being frozen, disbelieving, self-blaming, angry and sad. This was excruciating work, and of course Jimmy would never 100% recover. However, within eight months liveliness returned and he resumed interacting with friends and participating in life. A few months later he had caught up with his peers academically, was again playing sports and being invited to parties. His capacity to bounce back was testimony to the security he had developed in his early years. He knew that he had been deeply loved by both parents, and he expected to like and be liked by others. He did not expect disaster when something went wrong, but rather looked forward to novel situations, believing things would work out well. The secure child knows viscerally that they have a secure base to return to, which gives confidence, curiosity and a freedom to explore that insecure children lack.

Over decades I have consistently seen abused, traumatised or neglected children struggle with uncertainty. A shift in school routine, perhaps a temporary teacher, can trigger awful behaviour, a sign of extremely anxious feelings just below the surface, a fundamental lack of faith in life, little belief that new experiences (ruptures) are likely to turn out well.

Whether we bounce back or go under after a knock is 'overdetermined' by factors such as genetic makeup, early history, current social support and more. Children experiencing extreme stress in early childhood, such as abuse or early separations, are more vulnerable to later stressors (Haglund *et al.*, 2007), showing abnormally high stress signals, even as adults.

Equally importantly, a stress-free life is not helpful. We need to experience mismatches, and learn that these can be repaired. Children who come through mild stressors, such as moving home or parental illness, often are better equipped to deal with later stressors (Maddi,

2005). Too much stress, especially too early, does not help later in life, but neither does too little. Exposure to manageable difficulties can function as a form of 'stress inoculation' (Lyons *et al.*, 2009).

Being resilient includes finding hopeful possibilities even in major trials. This is not about superficially exhorting people to be positive and look on the bright side. Hopefulness is a deeply rooted personality trait that only grows with the right experiences. Trauma and stress adversely affect our pleasure-seeking and reward systems (Bogdan and Pizzagalli, 2006). Stress can lead to becoming aversive to exploration or social contact, while emotional security normally leads to happier, more confident outgoing children. Whether we are a hopeful Tigger, or a morose Eeyore, glass half-full or glass half-empty people, we react to a world we long ago learnt to expect. But as I know from my own eyeore-ness, and have seen in patients, this thankfully can change.

Molly again

This shift from despairing passivity to hope and passion was seen in Molly, who I described in the last chapter. She was the slightly autistic 4-year-old who easily retreated into a despondency she knew too well. She often attempted something, failed, and collapsed into a desperate heap, taking ages to recover. I had to avoid joining her in her ditch of despair, where she could experience us as two despairing people. What helped was standing outside her pain and demonstrating hope, doing what Alvarez (1992) describes as 'reclaiming' her.

In one session, she picked up an old-fashioned push-button telephone and pulled it towards the table edge so that it teetered, about to fall. My heart was in my mouth, foreseeing the phone breaking, the pieces scattering everywhere. In the past, if that had happened she would have collapsed forlornly. As it hit the floor, I gathered myself and managed to shout 'crash' loudly, trying to express the force, impact and shock, but also that this was manageable, even exciting.

She had been about to give up and cry, feeling that the phone, her play and indeed the world, was ruined. I retrieved a few parts and said, 'We can fix it, look', not in falsely reassuring manic denial but rather to model hope of recovery. I replaced some, and she looked at me, not quite believing that disaster could be recovered from. When I had repaired the phone, she wanted to start all over again, this time with an almost enjoyable anticipation of the crash, and helped replace the missing bits. One piece could not be found and again she was about to give up and I said, 'Oh where is it, is it here? Or is it here?' pretending not to know where it was but showing faith that it could be found. Hope was restored, she did not give up, and in forthcoming weeks this scene was re-enacted over and over. Soon it was her saying, as she searched, 'Oh I wonder where is it?' not copying me in an empty way but really identifying with hope, learning to keep trying when something went wrong.

One might interpret my intervention as defensively avoiding her painful experience of falling apart, but I became increasingly convinced that she needed someone to hold on to hope for her. I was allowing myself to be what Christopher Bollas (1989) described as a 'transformational object', evoking her as yet unrealised potentialities. When she nearly gave up and I said, 'Molly is not quite giving up, perhaps she can do it', this allowed her to persevere. Her subsequent attempts were followed by a triumphant 'Yes you did it!' from me. She showed pleasure and excitement, needing me to help her process hopeful and positive feeling states that luckier children take for granted. Soon Molly was doing this unaided, indeed becoming so lively that her parents worried that she was becoming 'naughty'!

Following a missed session, she arrived sad, also having trodden in a puddle and soaked her socks. She retreated under a blanket, crying for a long time. She tried to get up and kick a ball but rather pathetically missed it and collapsed again. Comments such as 'How sad you are' made no difference, nor even did saying things like 'You are very cross with Mr Music'. When I located myself clearly as a baddie she could rage at, saying loudly, 'That silly stupid old Mr Music, he went away, huh', she looked up, threw a plastic spoon at me and we were back in business, piles of toys flung in my direction, and she resumed playing. The rupture was repaired, more easily by now, despair replaced by righteous outrage. Such emotions have an 'outgoing' focus seen in more confident people, those who Davidson (2000) showed to have higher left-brain activation and a sense of agency. Indeed 'aggression' from the Latin literally means to 'move towards', a positive trait, the opposite of shrinking.

Some months later I was bowled over as the ditch metaphor was enacted before my eyes. She inadvertently knocked a doll she was playing with behind the couch. I expected a despairing collapse but to my astonishment she instead called out 'You all right down there?' She then said, 'I gonna get you out'. She found some string, leant over the edge of the desk, dropped the string down, and called out 'I comin''. She tied the string to the toy, climbed back on to the desk, insisting I hold the other end as she heaved the string with strenuous mock effort. She play-acted wiping her brow, pulled again and I joined her, triumphantly shouting 'one, two, three' and a loud 'YES' as she pulled the doll up. It was essential that I joined her and we heaved together. In the coming weeks, this cycle was re-played often, with slight variations, symbolising her identification with an internal 'life-giver' (Symington, 1993), who could pull her out of a psychological black hole, towards the light. By now a more resilient self, a robust internal object, was being established. She was being, as Alvarez (1992) describes, 'reclaimed' into life.

Research suggests that being slightly overconfident aids children's competence (Bjorklund, 2007). Generally, we become more realistic as we get older but younger children tend to think they can climb higher mountains, balance more balls, score more goals, are cleverer than others and they are adept at ignoring evidence to the contrary (Stipek and Gralinski, 1996).

Bjorklund (2007) sees this as 'protective optimism', not a defensive denying of painful realities. Such optimism is helpful for young children needing to learn, experiment and persist at tasks that initially feel too difficult. Bjorklund (2007) mentions another study where children were asked to predict how many of the pictures placed in front of them they would remember. Some massively overestimated while others were quite accurate. Maybe counter-intuitively, those who overestimated the most on the first round, who might seem to have almost delusional self-belief, tried out more strategies second time around and improved the most, their optimism encouraging them to persevere. Pessimistic children, lacking hope and self-belief, persevere less.

Children like Molly need help to develop a sense of optimism and of their own agency. In contrast, children of depressed parents tend to be more passive (Murray and Cooper, 1999), as do many traumatised or neglected children, whose confidence is often low. Obviously, there can be dangers in overestimating one's ability, but children like Molly run the opposite risk, of too easily becoming hopeless. Even though for all of us, reality, as grim as it can be, must be faced, too much painful reality too early is not in most children's best interests.

Shrinking violet no more

Good relationships, including good psychotherapies, are characterised not by harmony, but by continuous disruption and repair (Safran *et al.*, 2009). Molly would get a toy helicopter and crash it against the wall, and then place sellotape on the helicopter. I would naively say, 'You are mending it', as she said, 'plaster'. The same happened with a car and I, believing that my job was to identify with a hurt aspect of herself that needed repair, said things like 'Poor car is hurt and Molly is mending it'. Fortunately for Molly I was being supervised by the inimitable Anne Alvarez who pointed out my misguidedness. Molly was already over-concerned with damage, hurt, the need to repair and placate others, including me. Her hypersensitivity was such that often I only had to think about tidying up and she started putting things away, and at the tiniest muffled yawn she would worriedly say, 'tired'.

I learnt instead to emphasise the strength of the cars and helicopters crashing against the wall, not the damage and repair. Soon her crashes got stronger as I echoed her fledgling forcefulness with my own strong voice. Central to therapeutic technique is up- or down-regulating feeling states through vocal pitch, tone and rhythm (Greenspan and Downey, 1997). Meltzer (1976/2018) called this regulating the temperature and distance, sometimes speaking slightly more quietly than the patient, or more forcefully. As my forceful encouragement increased, Molly's bashes got louder, coming from an increasingly strong side of her.

She now zestfully removed the Sellotape/plasters from every animal and began to hurl them across the room. She said, 'Wanna help me?' demanding I join in, which I did, albeit struck by my inhibition in throwing exuberantly and wholeheartedly, as Molly now could.

This was a close shave. Without my supervision I could easily have confirmed Molly's belief that she had to be terribly careful, that she and others were basically brittle and fragile. I had been in danger of reinforcing the Molly who would shrink at the least noise, a Molly lacking in self-belief, who would give up in a desultory fashion at the slightest hurdle.

Molly never again put plasters on the animals, her version of the world now was more robust. I of course still needed to stay with how awful she felt at times, to feel her despair and be alongside her in her ditch. But she needed the strength in my voice, my conviction that when things go wrong they can be repaired. This included her needing me to 'mark' (Fonagy *et al.*, 2004) any glimmers of crossness, exaggerate such feelings, show that I could survive her rage and fury. She was changing fast. She carried herself differently, walking in a less airy fashion, her feet more firmly on the ground, often striding along with purpose.

Resilience and potency

I have focused on the development of resilience and hope, which have received surprisingly little attention in psychotherapy literature (Music, 2009). Good experiences are good for us, but so is learning to manage stressors. Mother–infant interactions are rarely smooth. Tronick (2007) suggested that good mutual attunement occurs only about 30% of the time in the best mother–infant relationship! It is the repair of mis-attunements that leads to resilience, when ruptures are not too catastrophic and repairs are good and quick enough. Secure children recover better than insecure ones from stressors because they have an overriding sense that things will work out, that the world is good and safe.

Resilience is marked by being able to face and grow from adverse experiences, not deny nor retreat in the face of it, as seen in what is called 'post-traumatic growth (Calhoun and Tedeschi, 2014). While we need to bear the difficult and dark aspects of life, as psychoanalysis urges, we also need to build positive parts of the personality. Many of us in caring roles are easily drawn to sadness, upset and pain, and underplay the positive. Others of course tend to minimise pain and the negative. However, we are advantaged if we can manage both sets of feelings.

To return to Molly, she was certainly becoming more hopeful and easeful. In one sequence near the end of therapy she looked up at the ceiling saying, 'I can see the sun'. I was assuming I was talking to the old Molly who did not do imagery, who was probably talking about a sun outside the window. She said, 'No, up there', pointing to the ceiling, and I realised, excitedly, that this was a sun coming from her imagination. I asked what else she saw and she said, 'A bird', and she asked, 'What can you see?' I said, 'A cloud'. This developed into a game full of imagination and pleasure.

Here was a genuinely nascent imagination. This rhythmic, reciprocal imaginative interchange and expanding of each other's gestures, was a sign of a 'true self' forming. Bubbles came next into her mind. She blew a pretend bubble in my direction, and I blew one back, thinking how genuinely bubbly her mood was, quite the opposite of the depressed girl I had first met. As one pretend bubble made its way towards her she said, 'I got a cheeky look on my face.' I was thrilled. Not only did she have a cheeky grin, but she had a mind capable of knowing, and of enjoying, the fact that she had a cheeky grin, a cheeky idea. I said, almost joyously, 'You got a cheeky look on your face.' She said excitedly, and with more than a touch of irreverence, 'I gonna burst the bubble.' I was left thrilled not only by her capacity for self-awareness, but also the impishness that heralded a newfound earthier robustness, a true self forming.

Chapter 4

Attachment and jumpy untrusting kids

Sadly, too many children who professionals worry about have learnt not to trust in adults, or in close relationships generally. They cannot 'bear the beams of love', which William Blake suggested is what makes life meaningful. Distrust and wariness are central to insecure attachment styles. In some environments it makes sense to develop an untrusting emotionally reactive way of being, but of course there are costs to this.

Rachel's adopted mother reached for the hairbrush, approaching Rachel with the loving intention to tidy her unkempt hair. This felt natural, what she had done with her biological daughter, what her mother had done for her, always an enjoyable experience. Rachel flinched and with cat-like swiftness swiped out. In the group I was running for adopters, Rachel's mother was in tears, at her wits end. Other parents nodded knowingly, sympathy abounded, such moments happened in all their families. Rachel's mother had not felt such rejection with her biological children and knew this was not her failing. When we offer love, and are rejected, it is so easy to feel self-blame, anger or both. The conversation centred around the 'attachment problems' their children had, which were much worse than they had been led to believe.

Why is attachment important for understanding troubled children? Indeed, what do we even mean by attachment? People talk about having 'good', 'weak' or 'strong' attachments, and we probably all know what is meant by such statements. This is the loose, everyday use of 'attachment', different from understandings from that very rigorous body of research called attachment theory. Still, these everyday terms do get to the heart of much of what we worry about in many children.

Our capacities to be close to others, to form bonds of mutual care and love, are the basis for relationships. We must feel safe if we are to trust, and 'bear the beams of love', and when we feel unsafe we close down, withdraw, defend ourselves.

Humans have a 'negativity bias', and some of us more than others are constantly alert for potential problems, predicting danger around every corner. Our negativity bias has been an evolutionary advantage. Any wild animal optimistically assuming there is no danger is more likely to become another creature's dinner than one who assumes the worst, even if nine times out of ten no real danger exists. At least pessimists survive and pass on their genes, unlike happy-go-lucky optimists. However, bad early experiences increase the negativity bias, leading to more distrust and less ability to give and receive affection.

Children calibrate how optimistic or worried to be, depending on how safe or risky their context is. Rachel's early life, before being taken into care, was fraught with danger, violence and unpredictability. She had to defend herself from a sadistic stepsister and aggressive stepbrother. We learn basic relational patterns early in life, including how sensible it is to relax or brace for trouble, to be dependent or self-reliant, hopeful or fearful, trusting or suspicious, tense or easeful. Children who suffer trauma are less likely to expect good outcomes or believe it is safe to depend on others. They often see danger when others see safety.

Freud (1920/2001) long ago described the 'pleasure principle', the simple idea that humans, like most species, move towards pleasure and away from pain. For too many troubled kids, relationships and intimacy signal danger rather than pleasure. Such expectations of relationships, our 'internal working models' (Bowlby, 1969), influence how our minds and bodies respond to new situations. However, often new situations do not warrant the old patterns, as seen in Rachel's response to having her hair brushed.

States of mind, such as distrust, suspicion and wariness, often develop for good reasons, but form the basis of insecure attachment styles. Tragically such children find unbearable what at some deep level they crave, to love and be loved.

Ambivalent attachment: Grace

Grace, 14, was the oldest of four children, each with different fathers. She was taken into care at 9 years old on grounds of neglect. Her mother had mental health and alcohol problems, quickly shifting from depressive states to manic highs. Grace kept safe by becoming vigilant of her mother's moods, including signs of alcohol use.

In this atmosphere of constant changeability, Grace became extremely watchful, an adept carer of her mother and siblings, working hard to prevent adverse moods. When her mother was feeling well she could be delightful, even loving, if somewhat over-effusive. The cost of developing such an accurate antenna for her mother's moods was being on almost constant high alert, anxious, needy, wary and overly solicitous of others. Her overly tuned attention to others also led to her being less in touch with her own thoughts, feelings and body states.

Grace's primary attachment pattern was insecure-ambivalent or insecure-resistant, with hints of more worrying disorganised attachment behaviour. Ambivalent attachment styles often develop in the face of unpredictable parents who a child needs to monitor closely, or even look after. I suspect that many of us in caring professions developed finely-honed abilities to read others' moods in the cauldron of dysfunctional families!

She was adopted late, at 11 years old, and a honeymoon period followed. She was initially viewed as 'caring' and 'no trouble', especially as she so dutifully looked after her younger brother. In her new school, teachers similarly found her helpful and pleasant. However, there was something unreachable about her, and it was not clear that she really cared about other people. Rather, her antennae picked up states of mind to keep her safe, not to develop deep and satisfying ways of relating. She often withdrew to her bedroom, staring into space, cut-off. She easily felt hurt and could resort to mild self-harm.

Grace was perhaps too easy a client, a welcome respite from my acting-out violent ones. In one typical session, she smiled nervously in the waiting room, looking at me longer than most people do and followed me. She was careful to leave space for someone walking by, looked down and smiled awkwardly. She was keeping everyone happy, including me, cultivating safety by ensuring that those around her were at ease.

At the start of one session, with her body half turned away, she asked, 'How are you?' I felt she had something on her mind and asked, 'How come you are wondering this today?' She hesitated, I encouraged her and she said, 'I thought you looked tired.' Here was a classic therapeutic dilemma. I in fact was tired, as I had been working away all weekend with no time off. As relational psychoanalysts point out (Aron, 2001), often patients know something about us before we know it about ourselves. Those like Grace with ambivalent attachment styles are often adept at picking up others' moods.

Often when my face had a serious expression she looked worried. I could fall into a trap of letting Grace be too easy a client, avoiding difficult feelings. People's 'expectations of relationships' are re-enacted in such ways, as we unconsciously 'nudge' each other into roles.

As we become cognisant of our own and others' habitual relationship templates in embodied ways, we can open the possibility of stepping outside of them, and slowly develop new relational skills. This requires a bodily and relational form of self-awareness, including bearing being placed into roles that can feel uncomfortable. Once we had got beneath the superficial way in which Grace made me feel good, I had to acknowledge that for her I was experienced deep down as another untrustworthy figure to be wary of. Being seen like this is a challenge if we like to think of ourselves as well meaning and kind!

Grace was achieving reasonably academically and had friends, yet often felt alone. She adopted 'tend-and-befriend' ways of keeping others at ease, her friends relying on her and not vice versa. She often felt rejected and hurt, such as when not invited to a party.

Following a split-up from a brief relationship she turned inwards, self-harmed superficially, haunting places where she might 'accidentally' bump into her former boyfriend. In therapy, breaks caused disquiet and she was often sullen before them. She was too polite to protest, the ideal client, almost perfectly punctual, and when slightly late she apologised profusely, fearful of upsetting me. Her preoccupation when late was to placate me, there was no thought that it was her who was missing out, or that I might be concerned for her.

Her unreachability suggested a self she could never trust others with. Donald Winnicott (1965) described people developing a false self to protect a 'true self', which remains hidden and undeveloped until experiences such as psychotherapy make it safe to come into the light. At her core, Grace felt alone, that no one really could know her.

Her comment about me being tired challenged me. She had accurately picked up my state. My temptation was to not answer, to bat her comment back, perhaps ask how she felt about me looking tired. In fact, I decided to say that yes, I was more tired than usual. Then I took a deep breath and decided to remark on just how very good she was at picking up my feelings, as she was with others too. I had to remember how Grace developed these skills as desperate survival mechanisms.

Grace's vigilance of my moods and her 'niceness' generally led me to feel slightly intruded upon. I sometimes experience 'helpfulness' of adult clients with similar attachment patterns as intrusive, overwhelming, even cloying. I think it was C. S. Lewis who said of someone that their epitaph should be: 'She lived for others; you can tell the others by their hunted look!' The term 'pathological altruism' has been invented to describe just this tendency (Oakley *et al.*, 2012).

I said to Grace how the world felt unsafe if she did not know what I or others were feeling. She looked relieved, leaning back, slightly relaxing. I said how hard it was to trust that I might still have her in my mind even if I was a bit tired, that she believed that if she did not look after me, or whoever she was with, she would be rejected or dropped from our minds. Earlier in the therapy she would have pushed such comments away, looking after me by saying things like 'Oh no, I know you are here to care for me', making me feel valuable, stroking my ego. This time though I got through, Grace receiving my 'beam of love' for a few seconds.

She began to cry. She had cried before, but this time the crying was different, deeper. Afterwards she looked more at ease and trusting, and talked about childhood memories. I had heard some before, but there was a new feel that had been creeping into recent sessions. She felt cross that she had wasted so much of her childhood having to look after her mother. The anger suggested some new self-worth forming, hope for better experiences with others.

She still had to carefully check out my moods, that she was not too much for me. Such patterns change slowly. In time though she began to trust more, letting her guard down. The sign that this was genuine was that I felt more at ease in myself, in my own body, which I linked to being less monitored. A new template of emotional relating was emerging in Grace, one that would never completely replace the old one, but might steadily take root alongside it, hopefully becoming her 'go-to' neuronal pathway through which she might filter more future experiences.

Silences and quiet stillness became possible in sessions, a sense that she could be alone in another's (mother's/my) presence, as Winnicott (1953) described. This was like a secure children feeling free to leave their caregiver and go off and play, knowing that, when needed, there will be someone there for them, so different from Grace's earliest experiences.

Such changes were incremental, with many backward steps. Luckily, we had time, Grace came for several years. Much of the work involved me becoming alert to how she tried to keep me 'sweet', such as by her suggesting how helpful, kind or perceptive I was! I needed to make space for her distrust, her painful feelings and dark thoughts, parts of herself she barely knew and was convinced no one else could tolerate.

Grace needed some backbone. We discussed in sessions how she accommodated to others, and was too compliant. We thought about how she might stand up for herself, and this very idea made her anxious. She was fearful of rejection, of friends withdrawing. In effect, she still saw and expected her mother's moods in those around her but began slowly to believe that other people's feelings were their own and not her responsibility.

She began to trust that it was ok, not shameful, to be angry, sad or anxious. She was internalising a newer more compassionate view of herself from her adoptive parents, from me and in time, from friends too.

One session just after a break I expected to meet the usual Grace, checking that I was ok, monitoring my mood. Instead she told me forcefully that she was upset that I was away. Another friendship had hit the rails and she had been desperate, telling me my timing was terrible, I deserved a holiday, but what about her? She knew, she said, that her feelings were irrational but she had needed me. In the past, this might have been said in a forlorn self-pitying way at best. However, this was new, an expression of anger, knowing that I could tolerate this. It was a huge revelation to trust that a feeling cannot be wrong or bad, that nearly always feelings arise for understandable reasons, can be accepted and often can be trusted.

Winnicott (1971) long ago understood that children need the full force of their emotions to be received, borne and survived by another. Only when our strongest feelings are managed and borne by others do we truly feel ourselves as separate, something that children in entangled ambivalent attachment relationships rarely feel.

Her mother would have crumbled rather than tolerate the force of Grace's rage, leaving Grace feeling too powerful, a cause of her mother's mental distress. Now she was having new experiences, feeling entitled to be an emotionally alive person with hopes and dreams, someone others would take seriously. She began to believe that others were present for her when she needed them, that she could relax her monitoring, forget about others' needs, experience the kind of trust we see in securely attached people.

Grace continued to struggle, and would do so into late adolescence and I imagine later. Yet she was becoming capable of embracing a fuller range of feelings, trusting that she was both loveable and worthy of living a fulfilled life. This was so different from her early hypervigilant watchfulness, her belief that her own feelings needed to always play second fiddle. These patterns had been appropriate for her early life but were no longer of use. Sadly, we do not shed old patterns like a snake sheds old skin – if only! But they do lose their power and new psychological skins form, new ways of intersecting with the social and interpersonal world. In Grace's case, a thicker, less porous psychological skin was forming, a less easily invaded one, a protected space from which to venture out into the world.

Adaptive attachments

All attachment patterns, including the most worrying ones, start as sensible adaptations to early environments, enabling children to fit in and survive. What we describe as insecure attachment should not be considered pathological or unhealthy. Too often I hear from adopters or teachers about behaviours that are experienced as intolerable, incomprehensible, even as 'bad', such as when children are over-reactive when there is no actual threat.

The beliefs and behaviours of these children developed to survive in families where being calm and secure would have been foolhardy. Amid violence and aggression, it makes sense to be hypervigilant and reactive, not relaxed and trusting. Damian was typical. A hyperaroused livewire from a family where shouting, reactivity and extreme aggression was the norm. At home, little love or psychological reflectiveness was present. I could startle him into defensiveness with the slightest movement or wrong look. My body was on tenterhooks much of the time, often tense and anxious. This taught me, deep in my being, something of how frightening the world was that he had once experienced.

He worked out my own reactive buttons and took pleasure in pressing them. He often pressed my fear button, and I was genuinely scared that he would lash out and hurt me. Harder to admit is how he pressed anger buttons; sometimes when I felt abusively treated I felt an inclination to show him who was boss, take him down a peg or two.

By 4 years old he had already been expelled from several nurseries. His anger and distress affected all in his force field. Damian was not bad, or mad, but his every moment was profoundly coloured by his past. His psyche, body, hormones and whole being was responding to the world he had been programmed to expect, even though in his new life these earlier skills were no longer helpful. Rather like the infamous Japanese soldiers still fighting in the jungle decades after the war was over, Damian was psychologically still living in a war that had in fact ended.

How selves develop

Children like Damian have not experienced being safely 'held in mind' so do not develop easeful calm. Why would they? As Winnicott (1971) had written about decades ago, the first sense of self is that which is reflected in a mother's eyes and face, and Damian's mother, by all accounts, was frightening and angry.

Newborns are primed to relate to people, preferring faces to inanimate objects. Babies of 7 months old can detect complex emotional states such as fear via changes in sclera, the whites of the eyes (Jessen and Grossmann, 2014). Even younger babies recognise emotions just by watching body movements, when faces are hidden (Zieber et al., 2014).

Recognising intentions and facial expressions occurs for good evolutionary reasons, such as enhancing bonding, fitting into groups or reading signals of danger. Such capacities become either blunted or overactive without attuned parenting. Children reared in emotionally depriving orphanages have less capacity to recognise facial expressions (Nelson *et al.*, 2013), with less activity in corresponding brain areas. Others, like Grace and Damian, are too aware of moods that might signal danger, but can rarely relax. They do not develop what Peter Fonagy calls epistemic trust (Fonagy and Allison, 2014), faith in adults and what they communicate. Instead we see epistemic vigilance. As an infant, Damian would never have experienced a world peopled by dependable adults, where he could thrive and learn.

What we call disorganised attachment strategies, being hypervigilant with threat systems on high alert, are probably the best of a bad job for getting by with traumatising parents. Damian did not receive what Elizabeth Meins (2012) termed 'mind-mindedness', that capacity of parents to be sensitively in touch with a child's state of mind and emotions. This is as good a predictor as we have of secure attachment, as well as of emotional regulation skills and executive functions.

Mind-mindedness is also a crucial skill for anyone involved with troubled children. The seminal attachment theorist Jeremy Holmes (Holmes and Slade, 2017) pointed to the similar qualities needed for good parenting and good therapeutically informed work. Like the parent of a securely attached child, a helpful professional functions as a secure base, helps create coherent narratives, is in touch with moods and emotions and can repair mismatches and ruptures (Tronick, 2007). Damian and the children in this and the next chapter had little of this.

The psychoanalyst Bion (1962b) famously described what he called containment, whereby a parent or therapist might take in and process an infant's experience and then give it back in a digested form. Parents read infant cues and respond, often verbally (e.g. 'Oh you seem so uncomfortable, I wonder what's wrong'). Fonagy et al. (2004) call this 'marking', an exaggerated reflection of an infant's feelings, almost hamming it up. Marking, like containment, conveys that an emotional state, such as anger or sadness, has been borne and understood by a reliable other. Infants and children who are responded to in such a sensitive and timely way, without too much parental anxiety, learn to trust that the world is safe, reliable and benign.

Other children like Damian have had to develop desperate coping mechanisms to get by, but at terrible cost. Children need what Damian did not get, an experience of their emotions being managed, contained and modulated, which leads to self-understanding, emotional regulation and a sense of well-being.

Disorganisation, chaos, rigidity and trauma

While anxiously waiting to meet Damian for his weekly session, I noticed that my heart was racing, my stomach was tight, my breathing shallow and my muscles tense, all symptoms of sympathetic nervous system arousal. Damian, as mentioned, had suffered violence and abuse and was hypervigilant, reactive, aggressive and 'wired'. His 'disorganised' attachment pattern arose because those who should be protecting him from danger were the ones perpetrating his abuse.

In his presence, I was often bracing against something bad happening. I experienced an anxious jolt thinking about him while travelling to work. I remembered last week's session, toys flying close to my head, confiscating scissors, Damian forcing his way into another staff-member's room on his way to his therapy. Sometimes it got so bad that I had to stop sessions and return him to the waiting room. He had run into the street, let off fire extinguishers and flooded toilets. The reception and ancillary staff all knew Damian well.

Damian grew up in a violent home with drugs, shouting and little calm. He was taken into care at 2 years old, and had had a string of foster placements. He had no further contact with his mother, who had never turned up for contact meetings. He was placed for adoption but no one came forward and at the age of 6 he was being approved for long-term foster care.

Much as neuroscience would predict, he was hypervigilant, expecting danger everywhere. In his presence, I knew I had to be careful, cautious, not move too fast and not vary anything too much. He was a whirlwind anyway but had been in a tumultuous mood since learning that he was not staying with his current carers, who felt too old to give him the care he needed. He was aggressive to other children, had few friends, was a playground bully and struggled to concentrate or learn. Despite being given 18 hours of weekly one-to-one support, his school doubted they could hold on to him.

In the assessment, I met a speedy, charming boy with an edge of threat. He could not really play, which would have required being relaxed, curious and open to whatever might happen next. Playing football, often a dreaded activity of therapists as it can be repetitive and not meaningful, was a relief with Damian, one activity he could engage in. He always wanted to win and made sure he did. He would score a goal, clench his fist triumphantly, yelp and eye me disdainfully. He would coax me into believing I could have a moment of glory, perhaps score one meagre goal to his hatful, but always quashed my hopes, leaving me feeling tricked. He was projecting something of his own horrible experience into me, taking malicious delight in making me the victim. For Damian, the world divided into victims and perpetrators.

In optimistic moments I hoped that by projecting his feelings into me he might have an experience of his feelings being made sense of. If he could see me bearing and making sense of being trickled, abused, manipulated, he might learn that they are manageable experiences, manageable at least somewhere, in me. In time he might start to believe that he could manage such feelings himself. However, at other times I felt that he was becoming addicted to the 'secondary gains' of enjoying power and others' suffering.

He had enough understanding of my thoughts and feelings to trick or hurt me, which is very different from empathy. Interestingly, when psychopathic adults watch people's faces or actions, their brains' empathy circuits are barely on (Blair, 2018). Even when they understand others' emotions, this understanding is without care, often to manipulate the other. Damian's brain might show similar neuronal activation, his potential for cruelty could be chilling and I rarely felt I was being treated as a person with feelings.

This is so unlike securely attached children who generally have high empathy, and get on well with peers. Damian lived in a frightening dog-eat-dog world. He had little capacity to reflect on his life, minimal autobiographical capacity, could not imagine himself into a future and lacked stories about his life.

It is easy to see why he was given diagnoses of autistic spectrum disorder, attention deficit hyperactivity disorder and conduct disorder. Yet such psychiatric classifications rarely capture the complexity of such children's issues, and maltreated children are often wrongly diagnosed (DeJong, 2010).

I tried to resist the deadening pull of constant football and when we played, aimed at least to expand on the characters. Didier Drogba and John Terry, powerful alpha-male Chelsea players of the time, were his heroes, ruthless figures with whom he identified. I described the feelings and character traits of these alpha-male footballing protagonists, which he permitted briefly before stating, 'Can we play properly now?' Moments of thought were rarely allowed. When he did not like me scoring he might say, 'No, I was not ready', and then at least I could talk about how upsetting it was when things did not go his way. Much of the play felt dead and sterile, interspersed with sadistic attacks and frightening outbursts.

In one session, on arrival he speedily took a toy, a female doll about the age of his foster carer, and began to destroy it. Aware of the possibility of an eruption I stepped back, took a deep breath and said clearly, 'Why on earth should you believe any adults care, after what you have experienced?' He continued to attack the doll, but less wildly, half glancing at me. I said, 'Of course you sometimes want to lash out and don't know why.' I had made a mistake, and he glared at me with menace. For kids like Damian just the word 'you' can feel accusatory and persecutory. I paused, trying to re-find my body, took a deep breath and began to talk aloud, as if to myself, 'Sometimes we can have huge jumbly feelings inside and we want to just explode, the feelings seem to come from nowhere.' He was still glaring, but the temperature had lowered.

I was trying to reflect back to him something of his experience, but in a digested form (Bion, 1962b). I took another deep breath, and noticed him watch me, and surprisingly, he took a deeper breath himself. He reached into the toy box and took some vehicles, including the ambulance. I had contacted a slightly trusting part of him, and he in that moment knew that helpful figures such as ambulance services exist, a precarious but growing belief in a helpful adult world.

More hopefully, he was now able to try to explain things to me, albeit in rudimentary fashion. He said, 'There is this boy,' as if I would know who he meant. I asked, 'Yes Damian, this boy …' and he replied, 'food all over his face' as he began to tell a very simple story. Small moments of hope crept in. He talked about how 'bad' he had been, probably told to do so by his carer. By now I could be slightly playful with him and we gave a name to this 'Cross Damian'. I tried to guess what 'Cross Damian' was feeling when he had got angry recently. He said, 'You sound funny' but relaxed, I think relieved that 'Cross Damian' might not encompass all of him, that there were other Damians, including a more caring one. It was important that I felt compassion for what 'Cross Damian' felt, rather than the judgment he was used to. Generally, he was becoming less reactive.

A few weeks later, during a football game, he turned the light on. As it flickered I noticed a glimmer of interest in him, and asked what he noticed. He said, 'The colour'. I said, 'Isn't that amazing, the room seems to change colour when you turn the light on.' He did it again, and looked at me saying, 'Goes sort of pink'. I said, 'Yes the whole room seems to change, and what is so, so interesting is that you noticed it, Damian, you have a mind now that can notice things like that.' This was the nearest he had been to genuine, open-eyed interest, to aesthetic appreciation (Meltzer *et al.*, 1988). He looked pleased, did it again and said, 'It makes a sound'. I said, 'Wow yes, you have noticed the sound it makes when you turn the light on.' I cocked my ear dramatically, and he repeated it. Then he said, 'It's like a star', which I repeated, enthusiastically noting how interesting it was to notice things. This is the kind of early attuned input that luckier babies receive, but Damian of course had not. Interestingly at the end of this session, for the first time ever, he 'helped' me to put the toys away, a shift towards cooperation and reciprocity. Similarly, school and home noted examples of increased thoughtfulness.

Damian shares similarities with many children who develop disorganised attachment patterns. Such attachment styles are not 'strategy-less' as we once thought, but rather highly organised in their alertness to danger (M. S. Moore, personal communication), leading to low self-regulation, easily aroused sympathetic nervous systems with propensities to flip from being controlled and rigid to extremely chaotic.

I found my single hour a week tough, but it was much easier than the challenges other adults in his life faced. I had the luxury of only concentrating on him, without 30 other kids to teach, housework to do at home or umpteen other kids on my social work caseload. My role was partly to develop a small oasis of calm, a place of safety in the room and in himself, which might grow, to which in time he could learn to return.

This oasis of calm is often called a 'window of tolerance' or zone of comfort by writers such as Pat Ogden (2006). I expand on this in later chapters. More secure children have quite a roomy, capacious window of tolerance, and it takes a lot for them to be triggered. Many maltreated children like Damian have a much narrower window, easily flipping into tense, angry states.

As his zone of tolerance expanded, and he slowly trusted it more, some reflection became possible, moments of calmness. He also became more likeable as he began to trust in the possibility of experiencing 'safeness'. I could say things like, 'It is hard to believe that I or anyone else can really be worth trusting or could care for you.' His play became quieter and increasingly included helpful and protective characters. While in this zone, he started to show small signs of secure attachment, such as empathy, curiosity, confidence, trust in others, belief that he could be cared for and even enjoyment of life. These remained rudimentary but were coming alive as real potentials.

Summary

In this chapter I have used attachment theory to make sense of why some children accept or refuse closeness, intimacy and affection. Children's emotional worlds develop in early niches. Through adapting to early families and contexts they form what Bowlby (1969) called 'internal working models' of relationships, which are then taken into other situations. In response to early experiences their brains become sculpted, hormones programmed, psychological beliefs formed and hearts set – all forming a deep groove. Attachment categories can explain how this happens, and within each attachment category there are myriad journeys whereby the capacity to trust and love, or not, takes shape.

Much of our job is to make sense of these patterns, in large part by becoming aware of how we find ourselves feeling, thinking and behaving with those we work with. We get drawn into the force field of whoever we are with, nudged into patterns of relating. With Grace, I was drawn into thinking I was being a helpful therapist who she trusted. With Damian, I found myself fearful, reactive and retaliatory. Making sense of such intersubjective patterns helps us understand who we are with. This in turn can enable new patterns, new ways of relating, new kinds of attachment bonds. With luck, such changes lead to turning towards not away from Blake's precious beams of love.

Chapter 5

Stuart

Growing an 'inner executive' and a mind to think thoughts

Introduction

In this chapter I introduce Stuart, who was 'hyperactivated', emotionally unregulated, restless and one of the most deprived boys I have ever met. I ended up seeing him for nearly five years, and witnessed many hopeful developments.

My first encounter was in the clinic waiting room. I was greeted by a world-weary late middle-aged couple, a salt of the earth pair who had fostered many children. Sitting close were two younger, cheeky boys, Stuart's brothers, appropriately staying close to their foster carers, suggesting a good attachment had forged in their three years together. Then I heard strange yelping noises and noticed a stringy loose-limbed blond boy with an awkward gait, all arms, legs and juddery movements. He seemed to be mimicking his foster father, making unusual noises and strange gestures. Despite his evident oddity, I warmed to him immediately, which I took as hopeful prognostically.

His foster carers told me some of their stories, but I had already read about the worst bits, including heartbreaking tales of chronic neglect, poor hygiene, terrible diet, sexual over-stimulation and exposure to violence. Stuart, now 11, had endured eight years of terrible neglect. His foster carers were struggling, unsure whether they could manage him.

I met with him alone to assess whether we could work together. He immediately started mimicking my movements, not sophisticated mimicry, more 'adhesive' (Meltzer, 1975), clinging to outward forms to hold himself together. This reminded me of Frances Tustin's (1992), view that some, mainly autistic, children fear they might 'liquefy' without rituals that confer a feeling of solidity.

While such imitation is a sign of profound unease, there is also something hopeful in it. As well as using mimicry to achieve some superficial sense of solidity, Stuart also wanted to learn how to be a person, and was trying to identify with adults he could learn from (Music, 2005).

Early days

Stuart had almost no impulse control. Watching TV calms most children but not Stuart, who was unable to sit quietly, but rather seemed almost inside programmes, moving, gesticulating, shouting. He would talk to himself, make odd noises, mumble and such behaviours increased when he was anxious.

He was also soiling himself, something seen frequently in fearful children with poor impulse control but also common in victims of sexual abuse. It was unclear what was behind this in Stuart. He was bullied at school and, not surprisingly, had almost no friends.

He had experienced shocking events, such as violence and inappropriate sexual behaviour. However, probably worse than what he was exposed to, were the needed experiences he was deprived of. Like highly neglected children I will discuss shortly, he received little of the attuned parenting needed to build a healthy personality. He and his siblings were basically left to bring each other up.

Unlike many traumatised children, Stuart was not aggressive or over-reactive. It is hard to explain how he escaped this trajectory. Often high levels of anger and aggression mask a lack of development below the surface, and Stuart's lack of anger allowed a direct view of his meagrely developed mind and emotional world.

His language was delayed, his speech peppered with odd, hard to grasp terms. He said, 'If I say H then I have a word. Catch got?' I said that I did not understand and he looked despondent. I tried to show that I would try my best to make sense of his words. He explained that if a teacher said, 'I want a word' then 'you can say H 'cos that's a word, or W'. He was presumably making a joke, but before had managed only something of their superficial structure, without the content.

He said, 'I am doing much improvements', seemingly an attempt to give an excuse for not attending, at least showing some intelligence! When I pressed him on why adults were worried about him, he said that he did not need help. I said directly that I did not believe him, and he looked aside and said, 'Well I lie', and then 'You got catch', which I think meant that I had understood him. He seemed relieved that I saw his need and was not judging him. I was hooked and intrigued.

I often made the mistake of using too complex sentences. Once when I did this he destroyed what he was making, and talked about 'neutral bombs'. I felt I had effectively 'nuked' his activity. Another time, I said something about his life before foster care, and unsure whether he had understood, I innocently asked, 'Does that ring a bell?' His response was to liltingly say 'ding a ling a ling', not mimicking me but rather unthinkingly associating. He was far from understanding the symbolism in 'ringing a bell'. Later he said 'mmmm', which I repeated, asking what he meant and he said, 'like a motorbike I think'. The 'mmmm' reminded him of an engine. Such responses are similar to what used to be called 'clang-like' associations (Shevrin *et al.*, 1971), often seen in schizophrenics who, like Stuart, could not manage symbolic language.

I thought initially that Stuart was defensively refusing to think about anything difficult. However, rather than not wanting to think, he lacked the foundations of a mind that could manage thoughts. Stuart's very concrete, almost clang-like associations were due undeveloped thinking equipment, his were 'thoughts without a thinker' (Bion, 1962a).

Much early work was about tracking thoughts, and in so doing facilitating a part of his mind capable of observing thoughts. If we started a conversation and he drifted off, he was relieved when I said, 'Let's go back to what we were saying before', allowing him to make links, joining thoughts together. These were the first stages of the ability to concentrate and self-regulate, of executive functioning.

Stuart tried to use Lego. He could scarcely make anything meaningful, but was pleased with himself, muttering 'never doing a thing like that before'. My attention on him enabled a new 'mind-growing' experience. Stuart need ordinary interested attention, nothing too complex, rather like how a parent helps an infant to make sense of the world When he began to feel attended to, he started to attend to himself, which again is how infant minds grow. Unfortunately, I often made overly complex remarks, which he thankfully ignored or brushed aside. As Winnicott was said to have suggested, a good reason for psychotherapists to say things is to be informed when we get it wrong, and in his unusual way Stuart informed me effectively.

Within weeks I saw signs of curiosity developing, albeit in Stuart's odd way. He asked, 'How come there are so many lights in Southend?' When I said that was an interesting question he looked pleased. When I asked what he thought he said, 'Oh I dunno I just thought that maybe, well, who pays and how if in a small building there are lights how many are there and maybe there is a generator or something under the ground, I don't know.' He was struggling with a half-thought he did not know what to do with. In another session, he told me about octopuses with huge heads that could get through little gaps and asked, 'How come?' and then 'and where did people come from, who invented them, was it the cavemen?' As absurd as this sounded, curiosity was definitely forming.

I was guilty, like many psychotherapists, of often working at the wrong level. When I said that he was really thinking about things, he visibly softened and breathed more deeply. However, when I linked his questions about where things came from to thoughts about where *he* came from, or even worse, to think about his father who he had not seen since he was 3 years old, he clammed up. This was several levels too complex for him.

Anne Alvarez (2012) has written extensively about how we must adjust our therapeutic technique to the child's level. With children like Stuart we must go slowly, not working at what Alvarez calls an 'explanatory level', not asking 'why' questions, or counterpoising one idea with another. It was huge progress when Stuart could even have an idea, even better if he knew he was having ideas. That was quite enough at this stage.

Self-regulation and executive function

As discussed, many traumatised children are in threat-induced hyperaroused sympathetic nervous system states, in which the brain circuitry involved in self-regulation dampens down. Much initial work with children like Stuart should aim to enhance emotional regulation and bodily awareness. Attuned, compassionate attentiveness goes a long way to help with this.

Trauma affects different children differently, but we often see issues loosely grouped together under the umbrella of poor executive functioning, such as problems with thinking, planning, self-regulation, self-reflection, working memory, concentration and relationship difficulties, all evident in Stuart.

Executive functions recruit our frontal lobes, particularly the prefrontal cortex, central to top-down tasks, such as inhibiting impulsiveness, executing plans, empathy and interpersonal skills. With children like Stuart we try to build both 'bottom-up' emotional/bodily ease, as well as 'top-down' frontal lobe regulatory and reflective executive functioning skills.

Here again Alvarez's thinking about levels of work is helpful. Most traumatised children struggle with anything too cognitively complex (e.g. using 'because' explanations such as 'this happened because of that'). They similarly struggle with statements that stir up emotions that they are not ready to manage, such as my mentioning Stuart's father too early. Many even struggle when we use the word 'you', almost feeling accused as in 'You are such a . . .'.

In Chapter 6 we see how children who Alvarez (1992) calls 'undrawn' need bringing into life, or 'reclaiming'. This works for dulled-down children, but overtly traumatised children need a different approach. Their primary presentation is not flatness, but being dysregulated and out of control. They might be undeveloped beneath the surface, as Stuart was, but their acting out behaviours need addressing first. Such work is less about enlivening, but more about down-regulating and calming.

Trauma and stress interfere with prefrontal brain circuitry and executive functioning, (Márquez et al., 2013), and regulating emotions is necessary to re-trigger self-reflection, self-regulation and other higher-order brain capacities.

The Boston Process of Change Group (2010), seminal infancy researchers and psychoanalysts, show that at the core of good therapeutic work is challenging habitual relationship patterns, what they call 'implicit relational knowing'. With a child who jumps when someone gets too close, because they expect to be hit, we are not dealing with repressed bad memories, and should not focus too much on memories of past events. Rather, a primary task is to develop awareness of 'implicit relational beliefs' that manifest in bodily reactions, such as lashing out or showing distrust.

Many abused children like Stuart are hyperreactive to stimuli, responding via what Stephen Porges (2011) has called 'neuroception', superfast and out of consciousness, amygdalae firing more powerfully at potential threat cues than more secure children (Kujawa *et al.*, 2016).

Creating a pause, a capacity for self-awareness and thinking, is especially hard for severely maltreated kids like Stuart. We were barely at the foothills of developing a mind capable of self-regulation and self-reflection. Eamon McCrory and colleagues (2017) at University College London and the Anna Freud Centre, demonstrate that the brain areas central for self-reflection, for forming narratives and autobiographical memory, are badly affected by trauma.

We can help develop awareness of such automatic responses by helping minds like Stuart's pause and reflect. As the great psychiatrist and Auschwitz survivor, Viktor Frankel, is quoted as saying: 'Between the stimulus and response there is a space. In that space is our power to choose our response. In our response lies our power and our freedom.'

Stuart had the hallmarks of a child with severe executive deficits. He struggled to hold two thoughts together, plan, concentrate and lacked self-awareness and self-regulatory skills. In psychoanalysis, we would say that Stuart's ego was scarcely formed.

What Freud (1920/2001) once called the ego might be thought of as the executive in executive functioning. A contemporary of Freud, Bekhterev (1907) in early twentieth-century Russia, found that damage to prefrontal brain areas resulted in losing the capacity both to plan and execute actions. Another great early twentieth-century Russian psychologist, Luria (1966), discovered that humans with organic prefrontal cortex damage were often disinhibited, impulsive, lacked self-awareness, struggled to listen to others or abide by social expectations.

This is also what we often see in traumatised children like Stuart, whose trauma affects such prefrontal capacities (Teicher *et al.*, 2016). Thus we need to work at the simple levels suggested by Alvarez, a view that fits well with understandings about executive functions put forward by Russell Barkley (2012) and others.

With what Winnicott (1965), called 'good-enough' parenting, most children develop skills in planning, purposive action, holding several things in mind and setting aside immediate temptations to pursue future goals. Secure attachment is linked to mind-minded parenting, which in turn is linked to executive functions (Meins and Russell, 2011), while stress, threat and fear inhibit these.

Stuart was on medication for ADHD, but symptoms of maltreatment are often confused with ADHD (DeJong, 2010), and both hyperactivity and poor concentration often originate in fear and anxiety. These are an aspect of executive functions that also are crucial for managing in social groups, hence why so many maltreated children struggle with relationships and become ostracised (Music, 2011). There is little space to build basic interpersonal capacities, concentration, empathy, kindness or curiosity when one's attention is focused on threat.

Children like Stuart can seem driven by what Freud described as the *id*, primitive unconscious forces nowadays often thought about in terms of subcortical brain processes. The *ego*, our 'executive', ensures that *id*-based impulses do not control everything. Thus, as Anne Alvarez (2012) urged, we must work at a simple level and try to put in place basic building blocks of a mind and self-regulatory capacities, before processing trauma or difficult memories.

Returning to Stuart

Stuart slowly responded to my attention, especially once I stopped speaking with too much complexity and realised it was counterproductive to put him in touch with feelings he had insufficient equipment to process. In one session, he struggled to connect a ball and string, eventually making a hole through the ball for the string to go through. I made a classic but unhelpful interpretation, saying, 'You really want things to be connected, like staying connected with your family, and with me in my mind.' He replied, 'You really are solving my problems ain't you?' I naïvely felt gratified by his comment, but in fact he then stopped the activity. My complex link had lost him. What I should have done was just emphasise that he had an idea, a plan in his mind, which itself was new. Perhaps next it would have helped to emphasise that he was concentrating and trying to execute this plan, and that he could now believe himself to be the kind of boy who could have a plan and act on it.

Interpretations linking string to connecting to his family were way over his head. I eventually realised this. He simply needed an experience of me paying attention, reflecting back what he was doing, commenting on his feelings, such as 'wow you are trying so hard' or 'oh no, it is really hard when things do not work out'. When I was silent for more than a few moments his thought processes became scattered or he gave up on tasks. My attention could hold him together now, starting to replace his reliance on odd imitative gestures, a step on the way to his own attention doing this.

Eight months into therapy he went to his locker and took play-doh, a ruler, pen, string and his exercise book and said 'Is this technology? I think so.' He talked about pepperoni and I realised as he spun play-doh in the air that he was making pretend pizzas. He had an idea of himself as a pizza man, and I talked about how interesting it was that he had this idea, and he looked pleased. He tried to make a box from the play-doh, failed and seemed flummoxed. To my excitement he drew a picture in his exercise book, a plan of what he might make, and then tried to execute this plan. Conceptualising a plan, and carrying it out, is a basic executive function, one that Stuart was now capable of. I knew by now that my main role was just to follow him, help his thought processes and his confidence that he was someone who could do such things.

He asked me about the holidays. Often, we psychotherapists too quickly link holidays to an assumption that we will be missed, and talk about how difficult that will be. I knew this would not help with Stuart, and I waited and he said, 'Oh that's another thought', as if astonished at having a thing called a thought. I excitedly said, 'Yes you have thoughts, a thinking person' and he said, 'Oh I have lots of them, millions, I've got millions of minds'!!

He began to draw indecipherable shapes on paper. I asked what they were and he said, 'Dunno, they just popped into my head.' I remarked on how amazing it was to notice that something could just pop into his head. He next excitedly said, 'I know what else popped into my head', and referred back to an earlier *Dr Who* game, saying 'I will exterminate.' He then said, 'They're, em, oh, they're . . .' and I helped him out with the word daleks and he said, 'Oh yeah, thanks, they're garlics' (!!). Interestingly at the end of this session he constructed a head, made a hole in the top and said, 'I'm going to put the brain in now.' I think he now really believed that you could build brains and minds.

In this phase we were constructing basic building blocks of a mind. This depended on him feeling sufficiently emotionally at ease and regulated. He was on the cusp of bigger leaps. A few months later he said, 'I'm not goin' to make pizzas, no, I wanna be a . . . [indistinguishable mumble] . . . they can ask for loads of money, you know thingy, yeah plumber, lots of 60 bucks a day.' I talked about how he had hopeful thoughts about the kind of person he might be in the future. This was rudimentary autobiographical narrative, imagining himself existing in time, as part of his own and other people's story. Many 14–16-month-olds can do this, when they start to recognise themselves in mirrors and use personal pronouns. Stuart at 11 was just learning.

Symbolism about emotions was also developing. While constructing something with Lego, he became aware of another thought in his mind. 'It is like my mum, piling stuff on top like this', as he placed several little bits of Lego on top of each other in a jumbled-up heavy mass. He then took a more solid piece and said, 'but with Paul [his foster carer] it is this, happier'. This was very touching. He was feeling more cared for. I talked about his new social worker. He said, 'Yah, he's a bit like you, bald head, but browner skin, a helping person like you, this is a helping house.'

Levels of executive functioning and therapy

With Stuart, I had to work hard to ensure that I worked at the appropriate level, neither too complex nor simple. Barkley (2012) suggests that basic skills can become building blocks for later ones. He calls the most basic level 'pre-executive', of early speech and language, memory and motor functioning. When I first met Stuart, he was struggling at this level.

In the next 'self-directed' stage we see symbolic play and rudimentary problem-solving skills, those often tested for in standardised executive functioning tests. Stuart was beginning to make some progress in these. This is the level where much initial therapeutic work needs to be focused with traumatised children.

Barkley's 'methodical–self-reliant', level, where we see more self-direction and the immediate environment being organised to achieve goals, is the slightly more sophisticated next level. This might include building constructions with objects at hand, which Stuart was now on the cusp of managing.

There are other levels, which remained well beyond him. These include Barkley's next, 'tactical–interactive' level, including the ability to develop longer-term goals, and to join with others to achieve what cannot be achieved on one's own. This means managing joint play, early team games, or bargaining. This is only Barkley's third level of five, but too complex for many traumatised children, like Stuart. There are more sophisticated levels, which were well beyond his reach, such as the complex capacity to follow abstract rules, morality and laws necessary to genuinely participate in communal life. Stuart, like many maltreated children, was far from this.

Stuart and memories

Many maltreated children are doubly hampered. They have less executive skills, are more reactive and quickly lose any tentative self-regulatory skills. We try to help children like Stuart become aware of their reactivity, to learn to insert a (reflective) pause, allowing emotional states to be mentalised and impulses inhibited. Then the mind (via the cortex) starts to represent experience, to generate thinking, transforming what Solms and Panksepp (2012) describe as 'fleeting, fugitive wave-like states of con-sciousness into mental solids' (p. 165).

We know from neuroscience and developmental research that we must feel sufficient safeness to be open, curious and in touch with thoughts and feelings. Stuart, in his unique way, was starting to feel safely alone in my presence, as Winnicott (1953) described. He began to spend time lying with a blanket and a pillow, albeit in a large sink in my room, not the most comfortable place, but for him a sign that he could relax with me, feel safe, the start of self-care.

In one such moment he said, 'You know what, I never thought of it but all the good things they were from my nan.' I asked, 'Like what?' and he said, 'Oh ice-creams and that' in a hazy half-dreamy way. He felt more at ease in his body and feelings, which facilitated the first good memories I had heard from him. Children like Stuart often need to re-find good feelings and memories before confronting difficult ones. He then drifted into a relaxed half-sleep. In later sessions he talked about having memories of his mother and father. He told me that he remem-bered them throwing things and fighting when they were drunk. He could just about manage to bear these memories, with my now benign presence, but only after he had found some reliable good memories.

A few sessions later he was more fidgety. I acknowledged his jumpy state, then tried to get him to tell me what was on his mind, something he could not have managed six months before. He surprised me by describing how he used to often see his mother having sex with his uncle and how horrible this was. He even mimicked the noises and I had the impression that these images often had to be pushed out of his mind. He now was developing a mind capable of processing memories, which previously were intrusive PTSD-like flashbacks.

Christmas was coming. He said that it was the best day in the year, that he had had three Christmases with his foster carers. He could express gratitude, saying, 'I feel safe now.' I asked about Christmases before and he described how his mother could not keep the beds clean and had too many children. He said, 'When I think of it, it is like there is a dagger in my heart.' Later he told me, 'In my new family, the dagger, it is like, fading away.' This was really touching. He even had sufficient self-awareness to say, 'I never talked like this before did I?' I said that he was feeling safely looked after now, and he repeated these words as if they had important meaning but were new to him, 'safely looked after'.

He added 'I like it here', and then 'I miss primary school', again retrieving some good memories, presumably building on the warm feelings between us. I asked more and he said that he missed the teachers, they were kind. He could trust in kindness now.

In the next session he placed chairs on the table and said that they were like 'all confused bits in a head', that the game was to put them back together again. I was amazed. This was uncannily reminiscent of Bion's (1962b) concept of containment. Here the baby projects unmanageable sensations, feelings and thoughts, what Bion calls beta elements, into the mother. She receives and digests these, rendering them manageable and meaningful with what Bion called 'alpha function', a metaphor for what happens in psychotherapy. I said that Stuart hoped I would help with the confused bits in his head, helping to make things less confusing. He seemed to relax.

I still had to be very careful. When disturbing things were thought about too precipitately he became distressed, and in one period his soiling re-occurred. However, by now I could help him calm down if I got the emotional tone right. He said, 'Yeah I do need you to help me with things like, well what I want to know is why my mum and uncle did all that, I need help with that.' I talked with feeling about how boys like Stuart should never have had to see such terrible things, things that were so hard to understand. He then described seeing his uncle being beaten on the head by a plank of wood. I was stunned, felt battered myself and spoke about how horribly shocking it must have been, he should not have had to witness such terrible things.

Later in that session he looked confused and said, 'I am starting to understand, it were my mum's fault, she should have some of that nicotine' (I think meaning the ADHD drug, Ritalin!). Later, excruciatingly, he mumbled several times, 'I wish I ... I wish ... ', and eventually said, 'I wish I never had a mum.' I again felt deeply moved, as if here was real mourning, loss for what he had never had and some incipient righteous anger.

Endings

I had seen Stuart for nearly five years, and when changing clinics three times I had fought to take him with me. It was not all positive. As adolescence took hold he became preoccupied with video games, and there were worries about pornography use. He was far from knowing the difference between perverse and ordinary sexual desires, but could at least start to think about this. Talking about pornography, he said, 'Yeah coz I might you know, not be able to stop myself ... a bit like snookered.' I asked more and he said that it was 'like the black ball, you never know when it will go down and that's the end'. Here seemingly was a mind now capable of metaphor. Soon he started a tentative relationship, which felt like an ordinary adolescent crush. He still had few friends, but there were a few children with whom he now got on with.

Nearer the end of our sessions he told me, 'I had another memory, we was in the bedroom and she [his mother] weed in J's mouth.' I said that that sounded like a really disturbing memory. He made a disgusted expression and looked away. I said that this was not something that any boy should see, especially with his mum, it must feel all wrong and horrible.

He then said, 'There is no point.' I asked what he meant. 'There is no point of life, no purpose, it's all a waste.' I talked about how sad it was that he had experienced such things. As I spoke his head dropped, and he seemed near sadness, even tears, genuinely bearing emotional upset rather than reacting to it. He was developing a mental/emotional container to hold such feeling states.

I repeated that he shouldn't have had to have such experiences, that he had needed adults who had his interests and needs in mind. He listened and asked,

> What is the purpose, I just had that thought, just now, there ain't no purpose. My mum, she had seven children, what do adults do for sex, how do they do it? I mean my dad and mum they just did it but there ain't no purpose. Do you know what the meaning of life is?

I was feeling very sad for him, moved at how he could be in touch with such painful feelings. After a bit he drifted off, and we were silent together for a while.

He then told me about being at home with his siblings, including his baby brother, 'all alone at 12 o'clock at night'. I said that it sounded like he had no one to think about him, which was sad and not fair. I asked where he thought his mother was and he said, 'Well you can guess, she was a prostitute weren't she?' He then said, 'They was both mentally ill. They never did think about me. She would leave us and go out to the pub, for *existence*, always going out she was.' He then looked pleased and said, 'That's cool, thinking ... no it ain't.' The 'cool thinking' suggested that he was pleased with being able to bear such thoughts, but the 'no it ain't' showed that he was not so pleased about *what* he had had to think about. Even young people as deprived and developmentally behind as Stuart can develop a mind capable of having thoughts and feelings, and profound thoughts to boot!

After nearly five years our work together was ending. In the last session, I said, 'Well this is it then.' He looked at me. I said, 'Relieved but sad at the same time', and he replied, 'Well that's a thing two thoughts together, not easy to do.' How right he was. Managing ambivalent, mixed feelings is one of the most sophisticated psychological achievements, one Melanie Klein (1946) long ago enshrined in her concept of the depressive position.

We looked through his folder at the work we had done together. He picked up a picture of a face on which he had written 'scared' and 'help'. He said, 'I growed up a lot innit?' He asked me what else we had talked about and I helped him recall many things we had talked about. He looked pleased.

Stuart at the start of our work was easily triggered but could not really know, except bodily, that he had difficult feelings. Now he had rudimentary equipment to process emotional states. He talked about his struggles with pornography, saying, 'I don't do it now, but it is like a battle, my body and the computer.' He talked about his hopes for the future, that he might even pass some exams. It was left to me to talk about feeling sad as we were parting after all these years, that our adventure was over. He said, 'You're right, you understand, I feel funny now.' My last sight of him was looking sad, struggling to get up to go. Some years later I tracked him down, gained permission to write about him and heard that he was involved in an organisation that worked with computer games, that he had a girlfriend and remained in close contact with his foster carers.

Conclusions

I have used my work with Stuart to show how developing emotional regulation is a precursor to developing a mind capable of thoughts. Poor executive functioning is a bad prognostic sign. We know that toddlers who struggle to inhibit impulses are less likely as adults to have good jobs or relationships (Peake, 2017), that impulse control and delayed gratification are the best predictors we have of academic success, that the lack of it is linked with many adverse long-term outcomes such as gambling, alcohol addiction (Dalley and Robbins, 2017), or worse, criminality and prison, especially after abuse-filled childhoods (Ford *et al.*, 2007).

The kind of attitudes that I have been arguing for in this book, such as empathy and emotional attunement, especially in the early years, lead to many positive outcomes. Children thrive when experiencing mind-mind-edness and parental sensitivity, including gaining better capacities for emotional regulation and executive functions. Even in severely maltreated children like Stuart change is possible.

Much that we do in therapy, or any emotionally attuned contact with children, is to facilitate the growth of basic psychological capacities, slowly and steadily. We should value input that can seem very simple, the kind of thing that most mothers do with babies. Ordinary attuned statements like 'wow what an upset cry, you did not like that' both regulate arousal and develop self-awareness. This was what Stuart needed initially, not the sophisticated depth-psychology understandings that I tried to impart too soon!

Securely attached children develop a felt sense of safety by experiencing attunement from reliable, compassionate reflective adults who can help them process their experiences. Children then internalise a sense of themselves as existing over time in the minds and stories of another. This is what happened for Stuart via his foster carers, therapy and school. Such children learn to feel calm and safe, and then to get to know their own thoughts and feelings. This in turn enables the development of an 'inner executive', helping children like Stuart participate in that most health-enhancing of experiences, being embedded safely in a community of people who care for each other.

Chapter 6

Left hemispheres rule, feelings avoided

Jenny and Edward

Typical of avoidant deactivated, attachment styles is a valuing of standing on one's own two feet, a belief that seeking help is weak, and that strong emotions should be avoided, particularly negative ones. Often in their families of origin deactivating attachment needs was sensible because vulnerability and neediness led to rejection.

My personal history includes being sent to boarding school at the tender age of 9, with no space for missing my parents, for emotional understanding or fragile emotions. I and many peers developed tough defences, psychological exoskeletons that aided survival, but left our needy, often desperate personality traits deeply buried, to be avoided at all costs. The psychoanalyst Herbert Rosenfeld (1987) described how in such situations needy, dependent parts of the self are denigrated, or alternatively, projected into others and attacked there. Commonly adults with a needy, ambivalently attached way of relating get into relationships with those with a primarily avoidant style. One person's neediness, often a man's, is disowned and projected into the other, where it can be denigrated, often re-enacting gender stereotypes.

The British 'stiff upper lip' upper-class personality typifies such avoidance, often reinforced by being sent away to boarding school at a very young age. Indeed some argue that this explains why many UK politicians are so deaf to young children's emotional needs (Duffell, 2000; Schaverien, 2015). This chapter outlines examples of avoidant 'deactivated' attachment styles.

Jenny

Jenny was 13, fair skinned, wiry, with a steely look. She was a challenge to work with in our nine-month therapy. She was cut off from emotions and unremittingly positive, in a way that felt unreal.

She was quiet, distant, but often diminishing of what I said, albeit in the nicest possible way. For example, if I tried to think with her about an issue, perhaps a difficult friendship, she would say things like 'oh that's normal', or 'of course', leaving me feeling a bit silly about saying anything emotionally alive to her. She seemingly came compliantly, because other people said she should. Not surprisingly I did not especially look forward to our sessions.

Before one session she gave me a placatory smile, sat down, looked away and said nothing. After a silence, I said that it is difficult to speak and she nodded. In her slightly distant way, she recounted a few events that seemed in fact quite 'uneventful'. When I tried to open things up I felt parried, as usual very nicely, Jenny insisting that everything was fine.

I asked again how she had been. She looked at me and said 'fine'. I looked back at her, hamming up a quizzical disbelieving expression, and she smiled. We had a narrative by now; she knew I would challenge her insistence that she was 'fine' and 'all good', that I did not believe her. I simply said, 'fine', a bit sarcastically, and she said, 'yeah fine'. I say, 'fine in what way I wonder', tongue in cheek, and she said, 'fine, just fine', a bit teasing, slightly self-mockingly. She laughed, and I joined in, we had made contact but were far away from real emotional relating.

Feelings had never been talked about at home. She had learnt to cut off from them. I noted how hard it is to come here, asking 'How do you feel I wonder when you are sitting here, like now, and do not know what to say. Do you feel nervous, worried, or maybe cross or embarrassed?' Her single word response was 'weird'. I asked in what way and she says, 'just weird', and I say,

> Uh huh. So, this is what happens, I ask a question, I try to inject feeling into this (I intone a strength of feeling into my voice, like an engine revving), I get a one-word response, and I feel I go like this (I make a noise like air coming out of a deflating balloon).

Something got through, she giggled, slightly relaxed, some colour coming into her cheeks. Needing to show respect for her defences, I added, 'It makes sense, you've had a lifetime of practising being bright and breezy, having no difficult feelings, there is little room for those in your family I know.' She relaxed, but also looked a bit challenged.

Jenny was emotionally detached and dampened down. I had to work hard to inject life into sessions, including using humour, which can sometimes backfire. I challenged her about having nothing to say about her week, good or bad. She mumbled about her friend coming to drama class. I asked about this and she looked somewhat nonplussed. I said, with as much feeling as I could muster, 'You really can't believe that I'm interested in you or care about what you feel.' A flicker of emotion ran across her face. I said, 'Feelings are a bit of a foreign country, especially the idea that yours might be important and of interest, to me, and others close to you.' She looked away, as if that was a bit intense, but seemed glad of my attempts to reach her.

I asked about her friend, what kind of person she was. She had to dig deep to try to find words to describe her friend and what was going on, how she feels and what she thinks. She told me that they have the same taste clothes, music and boys. I said 'and boys' and she retorts 'Justin Bieber' and 'he is amazing', and starts to describe him and I am drawn into something too chatty. Yet pushing her too much was counterproductive. Such small steps were progress, possibly the start of self-reflective emotional narratives.

I had to force myself to stay with any hints of difficult feelings because of the jokey atmosphere. With prompting, indeed prodding, she told me about having bad thoughts at night. I felt genuine concern for her, which I hadn't up until now, and asked more. She admitted sometimes having thoughts about self-harm and wishing she was not alive. I checked out how worried I should be. The danger of exploring potential risk was that she might experience me as unable to bear her desperate feelings. I had to be clear how she needed me to know just how awful she felt and not get too anxious. I found myself moved, unusually emotionally present with her. I said that, rather than things being fine, she had been unhappy and had showed courage in telling me.

She needed a breather from the intensity and repeated that she just wanted to be normal. I talked about how she partly wanted that, that I need to know the part of her that does not believe she can change. I wonder what that part of her might have to say. She found it hard to respond and I made guesses, saying, for example, 'Maybe it says don't trust that idiot, just rely on yourself.' She laughed, a slight flush to her face as if I was right but she was not sure if she liked it. She said that that voice was less powerful now. Soon we were back to silence, fiddling with her watch, her legs restless and I had lost her again. Perhaps I had got too near real issues.

She told me in the coming sessions about worries that everything will go wrong. I was struck by how riddled she was with anxiety, and realised it made sense to cut off from this. She said that everything must be completely tidy in her room, her bed had to be totally neat, no bits sticking out. She said, 'it must sound mad' but she felt more trusting of me. Here were her first revelations of obsessional traits that would feature later.

I said that always saying things are 'fine' is a bit like tidying everything up; maybe it is scary to discuss what seems emotionally messy. It was near the end of the session, enough for her today, and I knew I had to also respect her defences. She was fiddling around, jiggling her feet and swinging her watch, as if hypnotising me, smiling. I was struck again by how easy it was to get into a jokey flirtatious rapport, which pushes away feelings. I said that she had spoken more than she thought she would, which takes courage when she is not used to it.

Slowly she became more emotionally alive, and sessions became more real. The work with Jennie ended early, as eight months later she insisted she was ready to stop, stating that her parents were getting tired of her coming and that she does not want to feel like someone with problems. She tried to convince me that she was much better, being more assertive, managing many things very well. In some ways, this was the case. She had found a place in a popular group of friends, was doing well at singing and dancing, her obsessional traits had reduced, and her eating, which I had worried might become a problem, had normalised. I worried that she could return to dismissing emotional difficulty, to not talking about feelings, what Freud called a 'flight to health'.

Yet a new tone of voice, clearer, less false, gave me hope. She insisted that the reason that she had got better was her friends, not her mum, nor therapy! I worried that she was too determinedly happy, but also knew that she had had a good experience, and would return to therapy later if she needed it, which I suspected might happen. Certainly, symptomatically she was better, fuller in body, less pinched in her expressions, and able to tolerate and express more feeling.

In her final session, I asked how she thought she had changed and she said, 'I am not unhappy anymore, I don't mind mess so much, and I have a good appetite.' Her parents had in fact corroborated these changes in meetings with a colleague. She also seemed easier in her body. She said that she had grown up, was getting on better at home, indeed the whole family are getting on better, and that she was able to manage her friendships at school well. She went on to tell me about other positive things, such as dancing in some big shows, and a possible television game-show appearance.

She was most lively when talking about friends, especially a boy who she was now 'going out with'. She could show me that she was not finding it easy, he had 'blanked' her this morning, had not returned her last text message. I felt I needed to keep transference implications out of the discourse, although I did say that she might worry that she not will remain in my mind and thoughts. This was greeted with scepticism. However, she looked down at her phone, and I felt that she knew, and knew that I knew, that she had been powerfully affected by our work. She told me with some bravado that boys are 'not worth worrying about', but in fact she could let me know that she had dared to really open herself up this time, with this boy. I thought with me too. She said touchingly, 'I am a worrier, like my mum, she worries about everything.'

She talked about the difference from previously, when with boys it was 'dump them in a week'. I thought of how dumped I had felt in the early sessions by her denigratory avoidant attachment style, and how this contrasted with a young woman who, at least some of the time, was now in contact with feelings, touched by our contact, genuinely glad that she had let me in and trusted in my care. Of course, I remained concerned about her tendency to retreat under stress, to deny her worries, her pseudo-independence, obsessional features and propensity for having issues with eating. Nonetheless she had had a new experience of being with someone who could think about her and tolerate her emotional states, and had developed some capacity for emotionally alive and engaged relating.

Attachment avoidance and emotional deactivation

Jenny demonstrated how people can develop diminished abilities to bear emotions if ones attachment figures cannot tolerate them. By shutting off from needs they can remain close to caregivers without alienating them. The cost, as in Jenny's case, is disavowing aspects of the self and shutting down some of the richest features of human life.

In the test that catapulted attachment theory research into scientific more rigorous realms, the Strange Situation Test, a child with an avoidant style seems not to care when the mother leaves the room. Yet despite appearances, their heart rate increases just like the secure child who obviously is in distress. This suggests that they are feeling upset, at least at a bodily level, but that they have had to cut themselves off from such bodily signals. It is such faint signals that we are often trying to get people like Jenny to take notice of.

Jenny demonstrated classic avoidant attachment. She was emotionally un-nuanced, superficially sensible, insisting on being positive, and was difficult to make emotional contact with. The brain activity of those with dismissing, avoidant styles suggests a tendency to withdraw from rather than approach others, and be less aroused by emotional stimuli (Kungl *et al.*, 2016).

Interestingly, this in turn influences those in their orbit. Just listening to dismissive attachment-related discourses leaves listeners less interested in others' emotions, heightening activity in brain networks involved in social aversion (Krause *et al.*, 2016). Those with avoidant dismissing styles prefer to picture themselves as strong and self-sufficient. Such children under-report difficult emotions, and are less aware of having them. They have a falsely positive view of their attachment figures, one not backed up by their actual experiences and there is a profound divergence between what they say they are feeling (e.g. 'everything is fine') and how they actually behave (Borelli *et al.*, 2016).

Such dampening down of emotion makes them difficult to work with. Such children and adults are often described as having 'schizoid' defences, retreating into a cut-off shelter away from the world of powerful emotions and needs.

Iain McGilchrist (2010) has helped us understand this in terms of the brain. While there is no simple left–right hemisphere split between rationality and emotionality, our two hemispheres generally interpret and interact with the world differently. The left hemisphere in most species uses a focused attention, looking at detail, taking things apart and examining components, as in map-making, mathematics, medicine and science. We use our right hemispheres when we are scanning the broader environment, allowing uncertainty and curiosity. Our left hemispheres are more involved in logic and certainty, while new experiences are processed more in the right hemisphere.

Many of the central emotional skills needed in therapy, such as empathy and embodied emotional awareness, primarily occur through the right hemisphere (Schore, 1994), which is central to seeing others as feeling-ful and identifying with them. When patients have a stroke in parts of their right hemisphere, they can lose their ability to empathise or be attuned to feelings, and lose feeling for their body. As McGilchrist (2010) shows, the right parietal lobe is central to body sense, while the left hemisphere tends to treat the body more as more mechanical.

Interestingly McGilchrist (2010) suggests that the left hemisphere controls verbal discourse, with language, logic and linearity, even calling it the 'Berlusconi of the brain, a political heavyweight who has control of the media' (p. 229). The neuroscientist Michael Gazzaniga (2006), who researched split-brained patients, called it the 'left-hemisphere storyteller'. It has less interest in truth than internal logic and is an inveterate denier of unwanted realities. It also fosters over-blown optimism. Typically, many right hemisphere stroke patients with a left arm that no longer functions, deny this truth, blatantly say things like, 'I just do not want to move it today.'

We could barely function without our left hemisphere, it fills in gaps in narratives, helps make sense of things, but when not moderated by the right hemisphere, it merrily offers farfetched post-hoc explanations. McGilchrist (2010) and others argue that the right hemisphere acts as a kind of 'bull-shit detector' via its use of bodily sense, intuition and emotion. Antonio Damasio (1999) described something similar in terms of 'somatic markers', that *felt* sense in our body that signals things to us. It is no coincidence that people like Jenny, and Edward, who I will shortly introduce, are often out of touch with both their emotions and bodies. As Damasio has taught us, emotions are bodily processes.

As Allan Schore (2012) consistently brought to our attention, the right brain develops much earlier than the left, and is central for empathy and emotional regulation. Jenny of course showed many such characteristics, including hints of an eating disorder that thankfully did not materialise. McGilchrist (2010) shows how eating disorders come with left-hemisphere dominance, quoting a case of spontaneous recovery in an eating-disordered patient after a left-hemisphere stroke, suggesting that the disorder could only exist with an active left hemisphere. Dissociative disorders, McGilchrist suggests, are also marked by a left-hemisphere dominance, with a dissonant sense of being out of touch with one's body. Much of this can be seen in the intriguing story of Edward, who I now introduce.

Edward

In the waiting room, I was met by 12-year-old Edward, a wide-eyed, blonde boy, who was busying himself taking apart a toy. His father had a strikingly tight posture and superior expression, greeting me confidently, as if we were long-standing colleagues. In the room, he took the chair I usually sit in, with an expert air.

I asked where they wanted to start, struck by Edward's smug didactic tone. I found myself thinking that his neck seemed long, suggesting a dislocation between mind and body, as in James Joyce's description in the *Dubliners* of Duffy, who lives 'a short distance from his body' (Joyce, 1914/1992). He said,

> Well the way I see it, there are things that went wrong when I was younger and are not connecting with how things are now, it is simply a question of adjusting the circuits so that it all fits together properly.

Straightaway I was seeing impeccable logic, with little emotional substance. Viewing the body and mind mechanically is classic left-hemisphere logic (Mcgilchrist, 2010).

His father spoke in 'plummy' army-like tones, saying,

> Edward was bashed about as a little one, received bad treatment, mum was rather chaotic, me I'm much clearer. I am improving

things, I could do it all myself really, but he needs someone on the outside. I am of the Jungian ilk myself, more spiritual.

Despite a clear jibe at my therapeutic heritage, I was alerted to real trauma in Edward's background, alongside a primary attachment figure, his father, who managed life with exaggerated certainty and logic. Edward said, 'In my opinion you see, teachers do not understand and personally I think they are not worth much. The work I do, well it is what I was doing in juniors and we don't learn anything.' Edward had been placed in a special school for behavioural issues. His 'storytelling', certainty, logic and smug superiority fitted, as McGilchrist (2010) showed, with left-hemisphere dominance, alongside unwarranted optimism and refusal of uncertainty

He and his father tested me to see if I fitted as the 'right kind' of person. Edward displayed a badge, asking 'Do you know what that is? Do you understand about the scouts?' Soon after, his father, similarly, talks about being in the Freemasons, both taking pride in being secretly members of superior groups. Here were two classically schizoid people, very out of touch with feelings.

Father tried to describe his philosophy, explaining that he had been in the army, and liked to run the home on military lines. He said,

> With mum he could do whatever he wanted, but I teach him that he must do the washing, and we make the beds every day, and we wash and cook a bit too, and learn to iron, because we can be a little lazy and we will still eat with our mouth open but I say that at least he is trying now. It is slow progress after what it was like before, and at least we are starting to think now, and that is the point of rules. Tonight, I am taking him to the opera, we have been before, and you know there are not many boys of his age that get *that* sort of experience.

It was hard to get a word in edgeways. I was reeling at his smug superiority and rule-bound world. Father explained that he has set up a 'goodness chart' that 'includes everything such as behaviour, jobs done ... he is doing pretty well, coming out 83–85%, and if he comes out at 85% then the reward will be a holiday in Bali.'

I found myself worrying about Edward's feelings about his mother, who died only a year before, and asked about this. Edward said, 'At that time I wanted to end things', albeit speaking with no sad affect. He continued, 'and that would help me with one of my ambitions, because I would find out what really does lie after life, I would find out what other people do not know.' I felt flummoxed by logic that overrode all feeling.

Father told me that he would have an operation soon and would 'save' Edward from its gruesome nature by sending him to relatives. I wondered if Edward may feel worried about his father and want to stay in touch. Edward said that he would be able to tell, and father retorts, 'He is into vibes you know, quite intuitive and mystical', and Edward says, 'I can tune in to how he is.' Their emotionless somewhat bizarre double act again left me reeling.

I wondered if he had any feelings about not having seen his half-brother since his mother's death? He said, 'Well he is only 4, I have not had a chance to make a sentimental attachment to him.' I repeated 'sentimental attachment?' and he said, 'Yes, and I hope you will not be offended dad, but I think it is best not to make too much of an attachment because you never know what may happen.' I was stunned. This was about as avoidant of attachment as one could imagine. I said, 'You feel the same about your dad then' and he nodded. I tried to comment on his fear of closeness and strong feelings, but this gets lost in intellectualisation.

Six months later

By now, tiny shifts were occurring. In one session, he followed me with a big smile, whipped out a music player and started playing a track. I was feeling anxious about the noise, as he told me haughtily that this was a poor-quality machine, but good enough for school, his tone suggesting that it would suffice for 'plebs'. He turned it on and said grandiosely, 'Guess what? This is my favourite track.' I ask him to turn the volume down while noting that at least now I was someone with whom he wanted to share his precious things.

He said, 'Now, about the scouts, well I am going to give them the push as they are not up to it and I will not develop there.' He gets some toy cars and is on the floor playing games in which his military car inevitably controlled the others. I commented that he is pleased with the cadets but that the scouts in his mind seem inferior. I linked this with how he can make me and others move from good to bad very quickly.

This is too intellectual and had no impact. He could only be reached through subtler means, and he reacted negatively to any comments that had a hint of a critical edge.

My mind often wandered as he spoke in intellectual platitudes without emotional meaning. I said, slightly tongue-in-cheek, that he feels that he has it all sussed, and he nods, taking me at face value as if I have finally got it, and said that he thinks he really has, that things have improved immeasurably since he has moved in with his father. His car pulverised another, and I felt that this is what he did to my thoughts or comments.

I felt as if I had lost my bearings. I said, 'Sometimes I think you say something to shut me up, because my words feel threatening.' That was another mistake, especially the word 'threatening'. He could not bear vulnerability or uncertainty and needed to be 'top dog'. He said 'No', that he likes my words very much and agrees with them mostly. He went 'gotcha' three times to the other vehicles and then told me that he was man of the match at football yesterday. His smug victorious-ness left no gap through which I could enter his world.

I, feeling helpless, asked if he doubted there was any reason for being here. He agreed, insisting that everything is 'fine'. He returned to his game in which another victory was secured, describing what a brilliant strategist he is, good at sussing out enemies' weaknesses. I fell into the trap of making a somewhat clichéd 'you mean me' transference comment, suggesting that maybe he likes to suss out my weaknesses. He says, 'I don't think so, you see I think that we are both very similar. You analyse things and I do too.' He came to sit on the couch opposite me. 'Your job is to try to understand what is going on in my mind. And I sometimes try to wonder what is going on in yours.'

I asked what he thought was going on in my mind. Almost thoughtful, he suggested that I am very busy, with lots of work to do and must keep to exact times. I say more quietly, with some feeling, that maybe he thinks, even worries, that I do not really have enough time for him, that he is just another thing to fit into my busy schedule. He retorted, 'Not worried or upset, but confused maybe.' The atmosphere changed. Something had shifted. I felt I had made some emotional contact with him, and thought to myself how rare this was.

I repeated that he is confused by my busyness, noting that he had said a few weeks ago that perhaps I saw him as just a file, not a person, and that he wants to be taken seriously. I wondered if there was a part of him that thought that 50 minutes a week was just not enough. He nodded and said, 'Maybe, you could be right, if you get my meaning.' The atmosphere was softer, something had touched him.

To my surprise he tells me about a dream, the first one I had heard. He said,

> The clinic moved to America, but I just got a plane every time. But one journey, about five hours in, the plane crashed. I crawled out of a window. I had to choose four things to take with me and I chose a seat, which I knew would also turn into a bed, a pen knife, some cooking utensils and a torch that was manually powered.

There was a long description leading to him being on a desert island. Then he saw a girl, Grace, and they were there together for 15 years until a ship rescued them, amazed to see a flashlight from the island. In that time, they had had a couple of children. I think of the similarity between the names Grace and Graham, and am struck by possibly the first example of a need of others, alongside the omnipotence I knew all too well. I said that a part of him believes that he is very resourceful and can manage on his own, but maybe that hides his wish to have support, not to have to do it all alone. Maybe I could even help him. He dropped a toy and I stooped to pick it up and pass it to him. He said, 'Thank you very much'. I think we both knew that this 'thank you' was about more than the toy. A shift was occurring.

Nearing ending

Six months later we had set an ending date as they were moving to another part of he country. I felt both relief and sadness. As I collected him he said in his breezy over-familiar way, 'Hello Graham'. In the corridor he told me in a smug pleased-with-himself way, 'I have had a very good day so far, very good indeed, considering. You see, I found this. You may know, it is a travel card, I spied it on the pavement, and guess what?' He says, 'There was still £8 left on it, now that is what I call lucky. You see I can visit my friends now.' I was thinking about the loss of visits to me.

He told me about another travel card that his father had given him, saying, 'My dad you see he calls me Al Capone mark-2 because I am so mercenary', smiling in a self-satisfied manner. I found myself feeling irritated. He said,

> Well that is life in London you see, you have to be tough, that is my opinion, you see it may be different in other places, Devon for instance, it is different there. I have been there many times and I am very experienced. There you see if I dropped a card someone would pick it up and give it back, I know, I've seen it, and so when I am there I act like that, one adapts, but here it's you scratch my back and I ... no, he stops himself, its look after number one. Now the thing is that with this card I see no reason why I should not be able to travel here alone.

I was about to say something about his insistence on being independent, free of needs, but I knew now to be careful, not to sound critical, especially when irritated. I decided to take up the Devon bit of him, the Edward who can give and accept kindness, who even at times sees me as kind and helpful, who understood about people scratching each other's backs, helping each other. Surprisingly he relaxed and looked at me almost fondly. That was a close shave, I had just avoided returning to the battleground. Often it is important to take up the hope, the positive, not try to bash through their omnipotence.

He started to tell me about what I should do to be a better therapist, then softened and said, 'I think the other children you see would not be so challenging.' I said, 'Maybe it is easier to think that I am an incompetent therapist than to feel sadness at the ending.' He replied,

> No, absolutely not. You see maybe when my mother died I felt a bit upset for maybe an hour, but then I just went back to school and got on with things. I will not miss therapy at all. You see I aim to make myself like a machine.

I thought how true this was, but also that this defence was beginning to crumble. I smiled warmly at him, and as if picking up this shift in me, he seemed to mellow.

He then, to my amazement said, 'Well what I believe is that if there was a good God then why would he take my mother away in that way.' I felt this was heartfelt, something of his faith in life had been destroyed, and that he was also sharing how sad he felt at our ending. I knew I had to be careful about how I broached this. I said, 'Yes, that seems like a very cruel and sad thing. Endings are hard, losing people can be sad and you must hope that I feel sad at the idea of not seeing you in the future.'

He looked softer, younger. I said that he must wonder whether I will be able to hold him in my mind. I was softening to him too, by now able to see his arrogance and bravado for what it was, and able to feel for the vulnerable child with few other resources to rely on, bolstering himself by identifying with his father's superior ways.

Final session

In the waiting room he was listening to music, then came in readily, and at the door, as usual, put the engaged sign on. I do not think I ever managed to do this before him! He sat on his chair, got his box and took out his favourite military car, asking me whether he could take it. I confirmed that we had agreed that he could, that he wanted something to take to help remember our time together.

He said,

> Yes and this can go on a shelf and I will remember. I talk about whether he feels that I will remember him and our time together. He is surprisingly in touch, saying in a jokey way that he thinks that maybe he has been a bit of a horrible sod in the last few months and 'I hope you will remember the better things. Would you agree with that, Graham?'

He was looking at the car, saying that a real army car would not have the orange stripe, but that this one is for children so that they could find it again more easily if it got lost. I of course am thinking about whether he fears being lost from my mind, or me from his.

He started to explain something in his long-winded pompous way ('You see Graham, what happens is …'). I say that over time he has liked to show me how much he knows. He said to my astonishment, 'I'll agree with that, that seems fair enough, a fair comment. I have been a bit of a know-it-all. Oh, there are some toys there on the floor that must belong to someone else.' In fact, they were from his box. I say, 'It must feel strange that other children will be coming here after you have gone.' He said, 'Well that is life you know, I know that this place is not here just for my benefit, and that other children came here before and will after I stop.' I suggest it is not easy thinking that I will be doing something else at 10 o'clock on a Friday, maybe with someone else. 'You must hope that I will remember you, and miss our times together.'

He replied, 'Well I do hope you get an easier time of it next time.' I did not take up his worries about what effect he had on me. I was aware of a thoughtfulness I had rarely glimpsed. He said that at his new house he is going to get one of those whistle things that help you find lost keys. I said that he is maybe thinking about how he will find a place in his new life and not lose the good things he has developed, the keys to feeling better. He was surprisingly soft and quiet.

As the session neared the end he started looking in his box, playing like he used to do, especially with the cars, which he bashed about. He noted the marks that he had made on them, going through his box possibly for the last time. There was a hint of sadness. He said, 'Well that is life', playing a game reminiscent of the games he had played when he first came. He noted a mark on the bus, and said no one would notice that 'unless they were extremely observant like me'. I was thinking, but did not say, how he hoped he had really made a mark on me, and on the clinic.

He described how in the countryside he had trodden on something and mud flew into the air 'and my footprint will be there until the next millennium'. I said that he really hoped that he had made a mark, here, in my mind, a mark that will stay, that he has imprinted himself. He smiled, looking pleased.

I wistfully watched him playing with the toys. I then said that there was only a minute left and we better tidy up. As he put things away he nearly stepped on a toy, looked up and said, 'See, I do make mistakes.' It was a bit safer to allow ordinary fallibility now. I said, 'Time to say goodbye, last words', and he said, 'I will say that at the door at the end.' He put a few things in the box, looked around the room and said,

'Goodbye box, goodbye room.' I said as warmly as I could that I really wished him well in his new life. I held out my hand and he took it, placing his other hand over my shoulder, saying, 'Good luck and a happy and prosperous future.' I was feeling sad, tears welling up as I took him to the waiting room. His avoidance, so needed before he came to therapy, like Jenny's, had begun to break down, and a person with real feelings had started to emerge.

Chapter 7

Neglected children

Why it is easy yet dangerous to neglect neglect

Neglect's profound effects

Let me contrast my responses to two clients from a typical morning. The previous week, with 6-year-old Tommy, I ended with bruised shins, my room and psyche both battered. Tommy, who was shockingly traumatised, was a whirlwind, a handful for me, his teachers, social worker and especially his adoptive parents. Yet with Tommy I felt alive and interested. When informed of his arrival my heart beat fast, partly from anxious sympathetic nervous system arousal, but also some eager anticipation. When not being overtly bullied by him, I liked Tommy, he evokes warm feelings in other people.

In contrast, when my next patient, Pablo, arrives I note an inner deadening, I slowly answer the receptionist, am lethargic walking down the corridor, my breathing shallow, my mind dulled. Sessions blur into a grey expanse. My main intention is to keep myself psychologically alive in an atmosphere that feels robotic and dull.

I know that others feel the same with such children, but these are hard feelings to admit to. Therapists and childcare specialists are supposed to be interested, kind, empathic, not bored! In meetings, when his case is discussed the atmosphere becomes flat. His teacher and social worker struggle to be interested in him or give him what he needs for his mind and spirit to grow.

We know little about Pablo's early life. He was adopted from a South American orphanage when he was nearly 3 years old, his early environment provided his basic physical but not emotional needs. We do not know his age at entering the orphanage nor anything about his biological parents.

My reactions to Pablo are, I think, not untypical when we are with children who have suffered emotional neglect. Such reactions provide important information about their states of mind. This is not the kind of neglect that often preoccupies social workers, such as children coming to school dirty and hungry, or living in squalor. Physical neglect is very serious and too common, but the psychological sequelae of emotional neglect can be worse.

Such children may not have suffered violence, trauma or overt abuse but their prognosis is bleak. Worse than the bad things that happened to them are the good things that didn't, the lack of the experiences that lead to children becoming lively, curious or in touch with emotions. Think of the deadening sadness we experience witnessing pictures of orphans rocking themselves for self-comfort in bleak institutions, experiences almost too terrible to contemplate.

Like plants deprived of water and nutrients, neglected children's potential to grow and flower can atrophy. They then become flat and lifeless, with less cognitive capacity and emotional aliveness than more 'hyperactivated' children. Those who experience violence or overt trauma at least have had to develop enough liveliness to become reactive, unlike many who have suffered emotional neglect.

Returning to William Blake's refrain about 'receiving the beams of love', children who are emotionally neglected often have long ago given up on the spontaneous giving and receiving of love. Thinking back to the still-face experiment described in Chapter 3 (Tronick, 2007), when an attuned mother unexpectedly holds an expressionless face, her infant generally looks perturbed. They normally try to get their mother's attention back, perhaps smiling, pointing, screaming, using any pre-viously learnt interpersonal tricks. If these fail and the mother remains blank-faced, they generally turn inwards, resorting to self-soothing, such as clasping hands, self-stroking, staring into space or rocking. When other ploys fail only withdrawal and emotional shutdown is left, responses seen in highly neglected children.

Such children are a challenge to be with. In their presence we often feel dulled down, our thoughts become wooden, our bodies lumpen. It took me years to realise that what they have in common is not what happened to them, but what did not happen to them, a paucity of experiences that foster healthy emotional development.

I allow the term neglect to cover a broad spectrum, from relatively mild neglect, such as in some maternal depression and avoidant attachment, to extreme examples such as children brought up in depriving orphanages. Such children can be inhibited, passive and self-contained, with little ability to reflect on emotions. Often their capacity to form narratives about their lives is limited, they experience little pleasure and do not inspire hope, affection or enjoyment in those around them.

A crucial therapeutic tool is our embodied countertransference, our emotional responsiveness. Neglected children easily slip out of our minds. With Pablo, I often found myself thinking about mundane things like shopping. Our listlessness and lack of presence, echoing their dulled-down states, is important information that we need to own up to and bear, if we are to enter their psychological worlds.

Neglected children, having received little attention, turn away from their biologically inherited attachment needs. They then suffer what the child psychotherapist Gianna Henry called 'double deprivation' (Henry, 1974), not recognising any good care that is available to them. We also often see what Louise Emanuel (2002) called 'triple deprivation', as many are also neglected by professional systems. Neglected children are often the ones sitting in the back of classes causing no trouble, while the attention goes to the bright sharp ones, or the acting out, suicidal or aggressive children.

I am aware of the dangers of confusing symptoms and causes, and not all neglected children end up the same. Temperament, genetic inheritance and many other factors influence outcomes. Nonetheless there are enough commonalities to demarcate this group as needing specific understanding.

Understandings from attachment theory and developmental science

All infants are born primed to relate but this capacity turns off if not responded to. Pablo, described above, had turned in on himself early, giving up on relational contact, shutting down potentially interpersonally alive aspects of himself.

Infancy research shows how being held in mind and attuned to is growth-enhancing, leading to a feeling of agency and an expectation of interpersonal reciprocity. When things go well enough in the first year, nascent interpersonal capacities transform into sophisticated mutual understandings. From birth infants evoke reactions, can imitate and interact within social worlds saturated with meaning. By only 4 months infants can know they are the object of another's attention, even showing coyness (Reddy, 2008), and by 8 months can have sufficient understanding of other minds to 'tease and muck about'. By about 9 months 'joint attention' and 'social referencing' deepen appreciation of others' minds. Already the building blocks of empathy, altruism and mutuality are in place, but only when they experience what Anne Alvarez, after Colwyn Trevarthen, called 'live company' (Alvarez, 1992).

Such experiences, incrementally built up over the seconds, minutes, hours, days, weeks, months and years of a young life, are what gives rise to an internal world full of richness, trust and interest. It is exactly this that neglected children lack. Minute by minute, hour by hour, they have often experienced blankness, as illustrated painfully in footage of deprived orphans and accounts by researchers (Spitz, 1945; Tizard and Hodges, 1978). Too often they were left alone in an unpeopled world just when their brains and minds were ripe for development. While luckier children are held, touched, talked to, played with and loved, neglected children stagnate in a desultory world, remaining, as Alvarez (2012) suggests, 'undrawn' as opposed to 'withdrawn'.

A case example

Troy, nearly 3 years old, was placed for adoption with a couple with infertility issues. They had already adopted 4-year-old Alf, with whom they had their hands full. Alf's ambivalent attachment style meant he was clingy, demanding constant attention. With Alf, these parents were constantly involved and had no doubt how needed they were.

With Troy things were different. He was hard to warm to, in his own world, did puzzles and played with sand repetitively, not imaginatively and, most importantly, seemed not to need people. He could ask for things such as toys or food, but seem unbothered about who he was with. He would hurt himself but seek no comfort, and run off in supermarkets without a backward glance to his parents. On being reunited after separations he showed no pleasure, reacting to his parents as he did to strangers. His was an extreme variant of avoidant attachment, he had cut off from any felt need of others.

Troy's history makes sense of this. He was born to a single, depressed mother with learning disabilities, who barely interacted with him. He was taken into care at a year old, when neighbours alerted services that his mother had left him alone on several evenings. He was placed with an experienced foster carer who was looking after several children. She was efficient, the home extremely clean, everyone fed, clothed and changed. Troy was viewed as 'easy' and 'no trouble'. He did not protest at barely being interacted with, as he knew nothing better, so was left to his own devices much of the time. Indeed, his prospective adopters' first sighting was of him in a buggy with a bottle in his mouth. Apparently, such 'prop-feeding' was normal. He had had thousands of hours of learning to expect little from adults.

In my first meeting, the parents conveyed many worries while Troy wandered around the room, and shockingly it was probably 25 minutes before I realised that neither I, a child psychotherapist trained to be in touch with children, nor his parents, were paying him any attention. We had lost an idea of him as a human being with thoughts or feelings.

I began with dyadic parent–child work (Hughes, 2007) with Troy and whichever parent brought him. I modelled lively interactions, talking aloud about his actions, speculating about what might be happening in his mind, trying to demonstrate mind-mindedness. Any hint of an interactive gesture, such as him reaching out or looking quizzical, I hammed up and amplified, rather like I have described with Molly and Stuart. I worked hard to encourage the parents to spot these signs and mirror them back to him, so he began to feel alive in their minds. I suggested that each parent took time alone with Troy each day, since when both children were together Alf commandeered their attention and Troy, who seemed to need little, was duly given little.

The model I used comes from Selma Fraiberg's (1974) seminal work in the 1960s with blind babies and sighted mothers. Fraiberg helped these mothers draw their infants into an interpersonal world by pointing out barely noticeable reactions. Their faces might not brighten in response to their mother's voices but a toe wiggling here and hand gesture there were signs that the mothers were important to their infants. This encouraged the mothers to interact more and the babies in turn responded, becoming livelier and, importantly, more rewarding to look after.

Within weeks Troy's parents were coming with stories of changes he was making. I was moved, close to tears, when in a session I caught him fleetingly pointing at a picture and looking at me. This was 'proto-declarative pointing', pointing at something that he knew was also in my mind, knowing that we two were sharing appreciation of a third object. This is very different to 'proto-imperative' pointing where a child points simply because they want something. The intersubjectivity' (Trevarthen and Hubley, 1978) in Troy's gesture showed he was not on an autistic spectrum trajectory, as we had feared. We had shared what autistic children rarely do, a genuinely intersubjective moment.

His mother in turn became more interested in him and he responded to this. Some weeks later he was tapping the table and she said, 'Oh look at that tapping, you are anxious aren't you?' This felt miraculous. She had highlighted and ascribed emotional meaning to a physical action that before would have gone unnoticed. This is how infants develop a sense of being held in mind, and get to know their thoughts and feelings. Slowly this flat and cut-off boy became lively, interested and fun-loving.

Soon he began to play peekaboo, shrieking with delight when he was found, soaking up attention. To play peekaboo you must believe that someone has you in their mind, is missing you and pleased to find you. Troy now believed this. As Winnicott (1953) said, 'It is a joy to be hidden but a disaster not to be found' (p. 168). A few weeks later he stumbled, tripped and hit his head, but this time instead of getting up as if nothing had happened he looked up at his mother, his hands momentarily reaching out to her. This was the beginning of normal attachment behaviour, an expression of his need for her. We again were deeply touched.

Another sign of this was when I introduced him and his mother to a clinical psychology trainee who was to do play therapy alongside our family work. He anxiously cuddled into his mother for safety, showing appropriate attachment anxiety in the face of a stranger. Only months before he would have carried on unaffected.

After some months of play and family therapy he was remarkably transformed; indeed, his parents even worried that he was getting rather rowdy! He had begun to scream for attention, becoming rivalrous with his brother, refusing to be ignored, now a lively little boy who knew he had needs, could express them and knew they would be heard. He was also developing a capacity to develop narratives about his life and tell imaginative stories. He was young enough still for his mind to develop apace, as if a hidden 'true' self (Winnicott, 1965) was there all along, ready to spring to life if the situation warranted it.

At the point of referral, the parents were in crisis. Indeed, his mother later admitted that in those early days she thought every day about giving him up. 'Maybe one child was enough', she would say, and 'anyway it was probably not fair on Alf who needed lots of attention'. The truth was that they lacked sufficient warmth for Troy, and didn't enjoy parenting him. By the end we all felt pleasure, and indeed, love.

Troy was typical of neglected children in not evoking warmth in those around him. Neglected children often act as if they don't have needs, making us feel redundant, not evoking feelings of care. By the end the parents felt affection, love and passion for Troy, and would have fought to keep him. Troy's case was easier than many neglected children as he was so young, with much developmental potential. Nonetheless his story could easily have ended disastrously, with him experiencing a string of foster placements and growing into a cold, cut-off young person.

More on neglect, development and the brain

Neglect has profound effects on children's developing brains and hormonal systems. Without a 'companion in meaning-making' (Trevarthen, 2001) who can breathe life into their interpersonal potential, infants turn in on themselves. Then we see presentations common in the worst orphanages, staring into space, rocking, dead eyes, little responsiveness, symptoms that led Rutter et al. (1999) to admit that a large number of Romanian orphans seemed indistinguishable from autistic children. I have seen many children like this, often mis-diagnosed with Asperger's syndrome. One adopted former Romanian orphan rocked when distressed at the age of 14, struggled with relationships and took great interest in categorising and lists. Another's main interest was in memorising car manuals and shopping catalogues.

Bruce Perry (Perry et al., 1995) was one of the first to draw attention to how neglected children's chronically under-stimulated brains develop differently. Scans show that they react less to pictures of faces showing emotion (Porto et al., 2016), they show less metabolic brain activity generally (Marshall *et al.*, 2004) and less connectivity between regions central to social and emotional development (Eluvathingal *et al.*, 2006). We see decreases in cortical white matter (Sheridan *et al.*, 2012), atypical development of the amygdala and deficits in the prefrontal cortex (Maheu *et al.*, 2010), the seat of empathy, concentration and self-regulation.

The hormonal systems of severely neglected children also become programmed differently. They have lower oxytocin levels (Bos, 2017) and are much less interested in faces and emotions. Many also have lower levels of dopamine (Field, 2011) and underactive pleasure-seeking systems (Panksepp and Biven, 2012). Interestingly when stimulated, such as by massage, the levels of hormones such as dopamine and serotonin (central to feeling good) shoot up.

A helpful way of thinking about pleasure and seeking systems was developed by Paul Gilbert (2014) in compassion-focused therapy (CFT). Gilbert distinguishes between our threat systems, which come online when we are in danger; our soothing system, which leads us to feel calm and at ease when safe with loved ones; and our drive system, which moves us towards pleasure, excitement and appetites, such as sex and food. The latter is generally undeveloped in those who have suffered neglect.

Much psychotherapy is concerned with getting people out of the threat system, out of resorting to fight and flight too quickly and helping them back into the soothing affiliative system. Neglected children also struggle to get into the affiliative system but are less in their threat systems, as they have often not been subjected to frightening experiences like violence. Rather they have lacked good growth-enhancing experiences. This means they require a different therapeutic technique, one that stimulates pleasure, healthy excitement, novelty and hope.

Thankfully, change is possible. Children from depriving Romanian orphanages placed in good foster placements have been shown to improve dramatically compared to those who remain (Smyke *et al.*, 2014). They have better executive functioning, with its neural correlates in prefrontal brain areas, increased brain connectivity and exciting new growth of vital white matter (Vanderwert *et al.*, 2016).

In real life, thankfully, we rarely see the pure forms of neglect witnessed in very depriving orphanages. Most neglected children have some good input as well, and many also suffer overt abuse. However, they are nearly always avoidant and overly self-sufficient. Contrary to appearances, in the Strange Situation Test when their mother leaves them, avoidant children have similar physiological responses to secure children, such as sweating and faster heart rates. However, we seldom spot these signs of anxiety. They have learnt to cut-off from bodily distress signals, due to having parents who responded negatively to signs of neediness.

We often see something similar in infants of depressed mothers. When mothers are withdrawn and unable to interact much (Field *et al.*, 2006), children tend to be more passive, with less sense of agency, less curious or inclined to reach out to people (Murray and Cooper, 1999). Deactivated attachment styles develop for good reasons, but at a cost. The worry is we do not spot the issues as they can seem, from the outside, to be untroubled, not evoking worry.

Another case: Martin

Before a session with 10-year-old Martin, 18 months into weekly therapy, I already feel that typical flatness when the receptionist calls. I know this pattern by now and take a few moments to breathe consciously and get in touch with my body. Martin shuffles along, with a compliant smile. My mind goes blank and I already feel that anything 'alive' happening is down to me. I feel a less than proper therapist if I stay silent, but my verbal comments generally disappear into a chilling silence. I have learnt that to have any impact I must speak with a genuine 'feeling-fullness' and emotional honesty. I console myself that I have 'comrades in feeling' in other adults who have contact with Martin, most notably his parents and teachers, who also feel despondent around him.

Martin is the oldest of three, the others developing relatively normally. He was born some weeks premature, apparently with no organic damage, and remained in hospital for several weeks. At birth, his maternal grandmother was terminally ill, and she died soon afterwards. His mother was physically absent, but also depressed and preoccupied with looking after her bereaved father. Martin missed out on people attuned to his emotional states and was left alone too much.

He was described as a 'good' and 'quiet' baby, descriptions that often worry me. Presumably like Troy, he was 'too good' for his own good. He was frequently left with family and neighbours. Physically he reached his milestones normally, but he demanded and received little input. In nursery years, he showed little interest in other children, did not play in a 'make-believe' way, and was described as a loner. His parents experienced little pleasure from him, and he spent hours in his room in aimless activities. Children like Martin have little sense of themselves as existing over time in anyone else's mind, have not introjected a mind that is attentive to them and often show little curiosity or excitement.

I often had a shameful thought that I would be glad not to see Martin. I believe many neglected cut-off children engender similar feelings in those close to them, like teachers and caregivers. I suspect that cases like this, even when they get referred to services, are closed more quickly than others. We can justify this as the children seem to not care whether they get help, certainly do not ask for it and can be experienced as rejecting. It is difficult to admit to, but we can sometimes be relieved at the idea of not working with them, thus perpetuating their neglect.

The seminal psychoanalyst, Christopher Bollas (1987), invented the term 'normotic' to describe patients he said were psychologically 'unborn', often raised in families where their 'real selves' were not mirrored, with parents not alive to their children's inner realities. Bollas suggested that they have little capacity for empathy and are 'strangely objectless'. Another psychoanalyst, Joyce McDougall (1992), similarly described patients she called 'normopaths', lacking emotional aliveness or 'personal psychic theatres' (p. 156), with 'armour-plated shells'. She argued that it can take years before such 'rejected representations and stifled affects which surround this sterilised space become available to verbal thought and psychic elaboration' (p. 443).

It is striking how such clinical writings often have a despairing thread. The American psychoanalyst, Thomas Ogden (1999), argued that one's sense of 'aliveness' or 'deadness' is a revealing measure of how a therapy is going, and that therapists must be honest about their counter-transference. He writes with candour about fantasies of feigning illness 'to escape the stagnant deadness of the sessions' (p. 31). I certainly experience similar 'heart-sink' moments. Flat inner worlds, lack of imaginary play and little empathy make for unrewarding sessions.

This in part explains why we often need to develop a more active technique in such cases, aiming to 'reclaim' them (Alvarez, 1992), a deliberate enlivening rather than staying with the deadness. Otherwise we can be colluding with lifeless, obsessional or empty behaviours.

Sustaining thinking, empathy and internal freedom

Martin did not understand ordinary social cues. He looked 'uncool' compared to peers, was bullied at school but could not describe his experiences. He would say, 'I am a fidgety sort' as his legs twitched and his hands tapped, his body working at a speed that belied the apparent slowness of his mind. His fidgeting was his way of holding himself together, a self-soothing second-skin defence (Bick, 1968), compensating for the lack of feeling held in mind, or the internalisation of a good internal object.

He had no friends, although mentioned one boy who was as obsessed with trains and timetables as him. Cozolino (2006) suggests that in such patients, right-hemisphere emotional capacities are undeveloped, they are often logical, but with little emotional depth. When I tried to speak in my usual way, imagining his feelings, for example, my comments were brushed aside or ignored. I often felt myself enveloped in a cotton wool-like deadness. Sometimes I know I only spoke to feel psychologically alive. Bollas (1987) had written about how, with such patients, our words, spoken with meaning and energy, can become denuded of significance. Often such children do not so much ignore what we say, as not really notice it, irrespective of how empathic or accurate it is. Sadly, they lack the idea of a mind interested in them.

I often draw on the writings of British independent psychoanalysts Nina Coltart (1992) and Neville Symington (1983) and what they call 'inner acts of freedom'. Our internal mental work is the most crucial aspect of maintaining aliveness in such cases. This means being on guard against the trap of doing what looks like psychotherapy, but really is a form of pseudo-therapy. As Morgan (2005), a mindfulness psychotherapist wrote, 'the task is first and foremost not to be killed off. I . . . We are killed off when we are not present in the moment' (p. 141). This is easier said than done, when mind, body and emotions are so deadened.

Our shutdown states are in fact a form of role responsiveness (Sandler, 1993), 'emotional contagion' (Hatfield *et al.*, 1993), or mirror-neuron responsiveness (Rizzolatti *et al.*, 2006), rather than projections. Projection suggests communication and believing that another will receive one's communications. Paradoxically we need to be sufficiently empathic to bear their deadened psychological states in our countertransference, but without being drawn too far into their deadliness. Often empathy is the last thing one feels for them, which increases the challenge.

Martin had been reluctantly dragged to therapy by parents, unnerved by their feelings about him, including frustration and hopelessness, feelings I soon understood too. At school, he was viewed as odd, a loner, even 'stubborn'. In sessions, he would sit, staring compliantly. He obsessively divided up sessions, perhaps saying, 'I will talk about my dreams for three minutes, things at home for four minutes, play hangman for five minutes, talk about worries for four minutes.'

He inhabited a different world to any I took for granted. One week he made his list of 'things that happened this week', which included that his grandfather had died. I was shocked, and tried to show empathy. However, he looked at me blankly, told me some factual details about the funeral, but was far from feelings I wrongly assumed he would or 'should' have.

What helped was concentrating on what it felt like to be in a room with him, bearing my feelings, whether of boredom, irritation, wanting to shake him up, or drifting off. Once, feeling in a half-alive torpor, I concentrated hard on what he seemed to be experiencing and found myself feeling more sympathy. I think in response to my feeling tone he looked up and smiled, a moment to cherish, one from which some genuine relating followed. His smile seemed real, not compliant. At such moments my voice had more urgency, and genuineness, I was 'calling him back', 'reclaiming' him. I wonder what an MRI scan might have shown up in his or my prefrontal cortex at such moments, or what measurements a skin conductivity test would have revealed, but I feel sure that something would have registered in a way that was unusual in our therapy.

Slowly he loosened up, as I felt my way into his world, and I found myself liking him more. When feeling warmer, I could be more actively challenging of him in a less judgmental way. Sometimes my frustration crept in and my unsympathetic tones precluded helpfully getting through to him. When my attempts had urgency but not frustration, when I challenged him warmly, then real contact was possible. As I leaned forward saying, 'Oh wow, this bouncing leg stops Martin from feeling all nervy, but it keeps him from noticing that Mr Music is really interested in him', he looked up and his tone changed. Such shifts came from immersing myself in an aspect of his being that I found almost intolerable.

As he bounced his leg, I bounced mine in response and he looked up and awkwardly smiled. This was rudimentary but real 'reciprocity' (Brazelton and Cramer, 1991). As he stopped jigging his leg, and I did too, he looked up again, jigged and waited for me to respond, like the ordinary rhythmic to and fro that most babies engage in, which Martin as an infant had never experienced. It is through such reciprocity that a capacity for pleasure develops in babies.

Martin was slowly developing some capacity for managing more difficult feelings. It still made little sense to him when I talked, as I did too much, of breaks between sessions or holidays. However, when in a game, I enacted being suddenly stopped in my tracks and expressed mock frustration, he enjoyed this. He looked awkward, then laughed and in the next session he did a slightly wooden version of the same thing, showing a capacity for introjection and 'deferred imitation' (Meltzoff, 1988).

I have found that when such deadened patients start to 'thaw out' I often witness aggression and sadism. This can be hard to bear, yet I think expressing such unsavoury aspects of their personalities is, ironically, part of their lifeblood. Sometimes our disquiet at cruel features of the personality can lead to speaking in ways that stymie the genuine 'feeling-fullness' and 'aliveness'. As Martin became livelier I sometimes saw disturbing and sickly scenes enacted, such as of torture. If I revealed any hint of disapproval, his play ground to a halt. At times, I needed to speak to, or even for, the sadistic aggressive voice, empathically saying things like 'Yes, he really wants to beat him up as hard as he can, that's what you want.' As horrible as this was, there was some 'desire' here, some motivation and aliveness, some 'libido' being expressed. A big part of such work is encouraging 'aliveness', and as psychoanalysis has always shown, life is not always nice or pleasant.

Pleasure and enjoyment

Martin became more playful. He would sit behind a chair, wave his leg around, waiting for me to respond with an almost impish look. He began to show initiative, agency, but maybe more importantly, the beginnings of fun. I often heard an internal therapeutic judge saying that this was not proper therapy. Some emotions are not given enough attention in the therapeutic literature (Music, 2009), including enjoyment, excitement, liveliness and joy, emotions that neglected children experience too few of. Infancy research describes how babies love making things happen, whether making a noise by pulling a cord or making mother come with a cry or laugh. Rarely have neglected children developed this capacity for agency and enjoyment.

Alvarez (1992) in particular cautioned against mistaking a manic defence such as cheering someone up because we cannot stand their pain, for a genuine need to develop a capacity for enjoyment. She suggested that some children who jump on a chair and shout 'I am king of the castle' might be being defensive, but for others this could be a first experience of feeling strong and confident. They need this to be encouraged, rather than being trampled on by us saying something like 'you want to be strong but really inside you feel little and hopeless'.

Children when young tend to think they can climb higher mountains, balance more balls, score more goals and perform better than they really can (Bjorklund, 2007), and not experiencing enough confidence can be a sign of depression in children. Neglected children often have had no one believing in their capacities. As previously described with Molly, optimism can be a sign of emotional health in children, providing sufficient buoyancy to persevere with tasks. Most neglected children lack this. Earlier, when Martin had struggled to do something, like build a tower, he had quickly given up, but less so now. I actively encouraged him ('yes you can do it', 'no need to give up', 'wow, you are doing well') and he responded by developing some tenacity and hopefulness.

As well as lacking confidence, many neglected children have not been much enjoyed. In psychotherapy, we often privilege defensive systems, managing difficult experiences. Yet the 'appetitive', drive or 'seeking' systems (Panksepp and Biven, 2012) of such children badly need stimulating, via playful, mutually enjoyable interactions. We need to 'tip-toe up to pleasure' as well as pain. This is especially important for those neglected children for whom excitement can be confused with anxiety, which both use similar bodily systems.

When Martin smiled slightly, I could occasionally meet that feeling and respond, maybe with a 'oh yes that is exciting' or 'wow you really want to do that such a lot'. The trick was staying alive to faint, hard-to-detect signs of life, ensuring a tolerable level of excitement. I hate to think about the signs that bypassed me over the years because I was already too dulled down to notice them. When we amplify or 'mark' such signs of life (Fonagy *et al.*, 2004), they can become building blocks of lively mutuality. Neglected children need such enjoyable communicative dances to become more 'live company' (Alvarez, 1992). By the end, there were certainly moments when I enjoyed being with Martin, and he with me.

Conclusions

Neglect does not affect all children the same. Some can make do with less good input than others. Epigenetic research shows how some children are more affected by bad experiences, yet also more affected by good experiences (Bakermans-Kranenburg and van IJzendoorn, 2015). Maybe not all children would have withdrawn as Troy and Martin did. Yet whatever our genetic inheritance, all humans need some good, early, interactive care. We have learnt from orphanage studies how a 'deadly' lack of early interpersonal input can be more pernicious than overt trauma.

Field (2011) compared infants of withdrawn depressed mothers with infants who suffered intrusive parenting. Those with withdrawn depressed mothers were less exploratory at 1 year old, and by 3 years old showed less empathy, were passive and withdrawn and doing worse cognitively. Intrusion is bad news but is at least stimulating, whereas neglect is deadening. We start life with 'preconceptions', as Bion (1962b) stated, are born experience 'expectant', but if our 'evolutionarily expectable environment' (Cicchetti, 2010) does not materialise then certain capacities simply do not develop.

This group of children pose a challenge. With them we need to encourage agency and positive feeling and the paradoxical task of stepping back from a lifeless encounter in order empathically to be in touch with them. We walk a delicate tightrope between being there to amplify aliveness, but not being intrusive, between finding a way to foster agency and enjoyment, while being neither too manic nor seductive. To do this we must bear uncomfortable experiences but not be taken over by a numbing atmosphere. This is easier said than done. It is easy to fall back on rote routines, or too cognitively based ways of working, when we feel flat and uninspired.

Most neglected children I have known, like Martin, have not undergone complete personality transformations through therapy. They often slowly 'warm up', get livelier, slightly more real. Parallel work with parents and other professionals is crucial in ensuring that others too can identify and amplify hopeful developmental signs.

Sometimes parents, teachers and therapists might not be pleased that our work leads to children like Troy turning from quiet, dull and cut off to more lively, aggressive and challenging. However, what is most important is that some life is forming. Neglected children do not generally inspire therapeutic zeal, but unless we can find some passion and hope for them, then their prognosis is particularly bad.

Chapter 8

Bringing up the bodies

Body awareness and easeful selves

Introduction

Myra sat up from the couch, needing to see my face. She said, 'My mind is always racing, I can't relax, I wish my mind would give me a rest'. I was struck by her turn of phrase, particularly how she does not see her mind as *her*. Yet Myra has an extraordinarily fine mind, achieves well academically and has many intellectually stimulating relationships, all due largely to this mind that she does not see as *her*. It is not that she disowns her mind. Indeed, she relies on it relentlessly, absolutely knows it is hers, it is central to her identity, she is fiercely proud of it, yet it is not the core of who she *feels* she is. Often in sessions I sit beguiled by her sparkling thinking, yet I can lose touch with myself as embodied, my mind racing but losing awareness from the neck down.

With such patients I often find myself returning to Donald Winnicott's classic and prescient paper, 'Mind and Its Relation to the Psyche-Soma' (1953). Given leaps forward in developmental science such as neurobiology, these days clear demarcations between mind, brain and body make less sense, and Winnicott's, ideas are increasingly borne out. The innovative researcher Stephen Porges (2011) has put exciting scientific flesh on the bones of Winnicott's clinical genius, redrawing our understandings of the autonomic nervous system. Body awareness is increasingly central to good psychotherapy practice. Mindfulness adds to this, with its careful attention to immediate embodied experience. Interoception (Farb *et al.*, 2015), the awareness of the subtleties of body states and sensations, is vital when working with people who are out of touch with their bodies and struggle to self-regulate. The mind–body split, epitomised by Descartes' privileging the mental, has been costly. Psychotherapy mostly still prioritises the mind and thinking, *what* is said over non-verbal realms such as *how* things are said, despite new knowledge that emotions are whole body, not just brain processes (Damasio, 2012). The time is ripe to redress this in our therapeutic practice by working more directly with body awareness.

Psyche-soma, being and regression

In Winnicott's ideal world the mother's emotional holding and attuned sensitivity enables the infant to feel at ease, allowing, as he says, the psyche to 'indwell' in the body, giving rise to an easeful 'going-on-being' (Winnicott, 1965). Many lack the experience of safeness and calm that allows musing, just *being*, uninterrupted by what Winnicott called 'impingements', external or internal. Infants feeling stressed or unsafe resort to alternative ways of holding themselves together. These include what Esther Bick (1968) called second-skin responses such as muscularity, self-soothing, clasping hands together, stroking one's skin, staring at objects or using other sensations for self-holding. Some, such as Myra, use a precocious and overactive mind, sometimes called intellectual defences, to hold themselves together when it feels unsafe to relax or trust in the world.

Some British psychoanalysts influenced by Winnicott (c.f. Rayner, 1991) argued for facilitating 'regression' in therapy, where people can experience deeply relaxed, easeful states, reminiscent of what Winnicott (1965) described as the first real experience of *being* alone is in the presence of the mother.

The word *being* here denotes an experience in which the mother (or other) can be present but unnoticed, just like a fish does not know it is in water. The British psychotherapist Harry Guntrip (1995) describes this as feeling 'a profound sense of belonging, a being at one with his world which is not intellectually thought out, but is the persisting atmosphere of security in which he exists within himself' (p. 240).

Balint (1968, p. 142) described a patient who sat in silence for half a session and then began to sob deeply, saying that for the first time in his life he had been able to reach himself. Words, Balint suggested, can take us away from really being in touch with ourselves. Winnicott (1965) describes how people reach for thoughts in response to impingements, echoing meditation teachers who suggest that thoughts often come at a point of tightening or tensing.

Guntrip (1995) described patients who, when they could lay aside activity and thinking, contacted feelings of pain and despair that, when borne instead of defended against, led to profound relief and relaxation. In his own analysis with Winnicott, Guntrip reported being told 'you know about being active but not about growing, just breathing and your heart just beating while you sleep, without you having to do anything to make them work' (Hazell, 1996, p. 249). This too could be a comment from a mindfulness teacher.

Many people we work with, especially hypervigilant, traumatised patients, feel so over-aroused by external and internal stimuli that they never attain such relaxed 'going-on-being'. For them a successful therapeutic journey means moving away from an over-reliance on mental activity (Corrigan and Gordon, 1995) or bodily second-skin defences.

Paula

Paula, 20, came from a high-flying family, supportive financially but not emotionally. Her father was physically abusive and subject to fits of rage. He also crossed sexual boundaries, routinely examining her genitals 'for reasons of hygiene' during her adolescence. She described her mother as distant, tense and busy, and she rarely felt emotionally understood or held in mind, learning early to be self-reliant and untrusting.

Paula achieved well academically, but struggled socially. She needed to be in charge in sexual and other relationships. Not surprisingly, she was suspicious and critical of me. I often felt inadequate, kept at bay, too dangerous to be relied upon.

Her relationship with her body was problematic. Indeed, she described it as an alien nuisance. Her body though 'kept the score' (van der Kolk, 2014), and she often reported minor ailments. I experienced her as 'wired', her body taut with tension. Probably the intimacy of the psychotherapy context with a male therapist exacerbated this. She had few friends with whom she could relate intimately. She did though confide in her diary, writing daily in copious detail. While clearly helpful, this was also used self-reliantly, rather than trusting in a live human being.

She had since childhood depended hugely on willpower, control and rigid physical defences. Maybe more pertinently, she had had to override her body's signals about her emotions, typical of patients described by Corrigan and Gordon (1995), who rely on their minds rather than other people.

As often with suspicious, self-reliant clients, I felt dismissed, a bit useless, that little I said was helpful. Paula, who had never really trusted, was unlikely to start now with a strange man in an overly intimate setting. Empathy seemed to have no effect, nor did curiosity, and much that I said felt inadequate.

However, when I changed tack to enquire gently about her body states and sensations, I saw shifts. In one session, she reacted negatively to something I said and I noticed her hands tighten and fists clench. I said, 'Goodness, what I said was no annoying, the way you are clenching tight.' She looked at me and down at her hands, which unclenched as she remarked that she had not realised what she was doing. I asked more about the sensations, her urge to tighten, where else she felt anything. She could not easily answer, but seemed interested. A few minutes later she had tightened again. I asked if she had noticed, and what might have precipitated this. She was surprised at the automaticity of her actions. Marion Milner, so gifted in her use of sensory awareness, long ago described a 'contracted' attitude to life, closing up at signs of threat, just as a sea anemone might (Milner, 1936). Paula did this more easily than most.

In the forthcoming weeks, she reported noticing tensing up in various situations. As she spoke about what made her anxious, or when I noticed a negative response to something I said, I would ask what was happening in her body, such as holding her breath. She was increasingly interested in this, noticing how she was holding her body tightly, or pacing agitatedly during mundane tasks such as waiting for the kettle. Such noticing allowed her to relax the holding, albeit momentarily. Of course, given her history and my gender, I needed to be extremely cautious about focusing on bodily issues.

Securely attached children, who generally have experienced sensitive attunement, tend automatically to develop an ability to self-regulate.

Experiences of being understood are internalised, allowing self-awareness, including of body signals. Becoming consciously aware of bodily processes, as Paula was, is only a start and in time such self-regulatory skills can become automatic procedural processes.

Damasio (2012) suggests that consciousness enables us to deliberately act in ways that can become second nature. In therapy we are building executive capacities, what Freud called the ego, which inhibits impulses, drives or urges, something that eventually happens automatically, out of consciousness. Such skills often start with tracking basic body sensations, both in the patient and in the therapist's embodied countertransference.

Vagus nerves and the autonomic nervous system

Porges (2011) describes a branch of the autonomic nervous system seen in mammals, and in increasingly complex form in humans, which is central to easeful 'going-on-being'. A sophisticated myelinated (ventral) branch of our vagus nerve (the 'smart vagus') connects our brain stem, heart, stomach and other viscera, as well as our facial muscles. This is active in bonding, social communication, recognising faces and expressing emotions. It fires alongside feelings such as that warm glow in our chests when with someone we love, when feeling gratitude or deep ease.

This system stops working, or as Porges says, the vagal brake comes off, in anxiety, fear or threat, when our sympathetic nervous system kicks in, including fight–flight responses. Then we experience increased heart rates, sweating, quicker breathing, dilation of pupils and inhibited digestion. We need this arousal system at times but following trauma we flip too quickly into such dysregulated states.

Mick was typical, hyperactive in school, and aggressive at the slightest hint of insult. He had lived his ten years in a neglectful unpredictable environment, with violence, drugs, few boundaries and little sensitive caregiving. He expected a dangerous world, one where it is unsafe to be vulnerable or trusting, where one had to get one's revenge in first. These were good survival strategies in his early environment, but were not working since being fostered. Mick's sympathetic nervous system seemed almost constantly aroused, his breathing shallow, his body braced for action, heart rate fast, presumably stress hormones coursing through his body.

Effective psychotherapy for trauma enhances activity in top-down brain circuitry central to executive functioning, (Márquez *et al.*, 2013), tuning down the primitive subcortical areas central to fear. This happens by facilitating feelings of safety, calm and openness to others. This 'rest and digest' aspect of the parasympathetic nervous system opens the possibility of emotional closeness, teamwork and cooperation. Physiologically it leads to lower heart rate and blood pressure, more relaxed states, deeper breathing, enhanced digestive and immune systems, all advantageous in safe environments

Such traits are easily measured via heart-rate variability, the variation in intervals between heartbeats or respiratory sinus arrhythmia (RSA). People with more heart-rate variability have higher vagal tone, which comes with being more relaxed and open. Low vagal tone is linked with many poor physical and mental health outcomes across the lifespan (Pakulak *et al.*, 2018). Poor parenting and maltreatment, for example, lead to low vagal tone (Rudd *et al.*, 2017).

Better vagal tone comes with being more calm after stressful triggers and better repair of interactions that go awry, even in infants (Provenzi *et al.*, 2015), and is also linked with compassionate states of mind (Stellar *et al.*, 2015). Generally, people with high vagal tone experience more emotional well-being on many measures, including doing better cognitively and having fewer social problems (Graziano and Derefinko, 2013). While vagal tone is powerfully affected by early experiences, practices such as mindfulness, psychotherapy, diet and breathing exercises can change it for the better.

While I have concentrated more on dysregulated and over-aroused patients. Porges' theory makes really important contributions to understanding patients who rely on primitive freeze, numbing and dissociated states, which I take up in the next chapter. Such shutdown states of immobilisation are resorted to when not only the smart vagus system but also the sympathetic nervous system's fight–flight systems have failed. Then humans, like all mammals, turn to the least sophisticated branch of our autonomic nervous system, the dorsal vagus branch, which we share with our most primitive premammalian ancestors, leading to numbness, metabolic shutdown and 'playing dead'. Such dissociative states of mind are in many ways the most worrying of all.

I believe that in psychotherapy we are helping to reconfigure nervous systems so that the smart vagus is firing and people can feel more at ease. This is very like Winnicott's descriptions of people moving into states of 'going-on-being', so different to precocious overly busy minds, or agitated bodies.

Examples

With Mick, Paula and others, alongside a new belief that they could be held in mind, came more ability to relax and be in the moment. In Paula's case, long periods of silence emerged during which I struggled to trust that my quiet inactivity could still be called psychotherapy! There were periods of deep contact accompanied by painful emotions, maybe like the classic cases of regression that Winnicott and Guntrip described.

In Mick's case, as is common for his age, I did not see overt outpourings of grief or mourning for the life he did not have. I did see him become stiller, less hypervigilant and manic. He indulged in quieter play, would make dens for himself, covering himself with a blanket, making me wait quietly for long periods. He too was learning about 'being alone in the presence of', learning to trust stillness, even basking in it.

Many such dysregulated patients are very out of touch with what is going on inside their own skins. Enhancing our own body awareness helps us be with others more meaningfully. In one session with Mick I found myself feeling tense and anxious, worried that he would do something unsafe like climb a high cupboard or throw something dangerously. My heart was in my mouth, my body tight and breathing shallow. Just the process of noticing this led to my body relaxing, allowing me to take on a more self-assured and easeful stance, stepping outside of a potentially combative enactment (Aron, 2001).

Another time Mick was again restless and jumpy, and I was becoming edgy. Noticing my tension, I took a deep breath, trying to stay with my feeling. When I looked up again he was calmly drawing. Whether my simple act of self-regulation had an effect would be hard to prove, but we know how people non-consciously resonate with other's body states, such as via mirror-neurons (Rizzolatti *et al.*, 2006).

Often, I would simply echo Mick's feelings, letting him know they were understood. He developed confidence that this would happen and began to regulate such feelings for himself. Feeling understood can bring relief and relaxation without the therapist being explicit about what is happening.

We can take a step further and help patients to consciously become aware of what is going on physiologically, as I described with Paula. Bringing awareness to tension, for example, can allow a relaxing. Practice and habit increase such self-regulatory awareness, training our interoceptive self-awareness muscles. Such new psychic muscles are in effect what psychoanalysis thinks of as good internal objects, derived from identification with a 'noticing other' (object), enhancing bodily states of softness, ease and relaxation.

Sometimes insight can make a difference of course. In one session Paula was raging at her new boyfriend's behaviour, and I simply suggested, based on understanding that had developed between us, that her provocative actions might have given him cause to feel jealous. This is the bread and butter of much therapy and made no reference to bodily states. Paula said something like 'oh yeah', raised her eyebrows, smiled, and her whole being calmed down. Here insight alone led to bodily relaxation.

At other times, nothing I said made much difference, and she remained agitated, angry or dysregulated. Possibly I lacked the skill to find the correct calming psychological interpretation, although once people get very aroused they can become hard to reach with interpretations. Alvarez's (2012) innovative thinking has pushed us to carefully consider our therapeutic technique, in particular, whether we might work at too cognitive a level with certain patients. In therapy with overtly abused patients I often find it necessary to work at a more psychophysiological level, such as down-regulating powerful emotions and managing over-arousal.

Asking questions with genuine curiosity about bodily experiences can unleash profound associations. In one session, Paula was talking angrily about someone who had upset her. I was struck by the unusual way that she started to rub her cheeks, which had reddened. I asked what was happening, what she was feeling in her face. She falteringly told me how her father would slap her on her cheeks when she was getting upset. This brought up an extraordinary stream of material about childhood experiences with her father. These would never have come to light had I not enquired about how she was rubbing her cheeks, which had reddened as if her cheeks were the medium for the expression of consciously forgotten but bodily remembered childhood experiences.

Sometimes we can actively guide patients to become more aware of bodily states. This can be relatively non-directive, such as wondering if it is ok to stop holding tightly against tears, which is tantamount to giving someone permission to cry. For example, when Paula was near sadness but bracing against this, I suggested she might breathe more deeply, showing my trust that we could manage her feelings together.

The step further, possibly too far for some, is actively encouraging awareness of body states by offering some instruction. For a few years I met with senior psychoanalytic psychotherapy colleagues who shared an interest in both brain science and mindfulness. We had all benefitted from our own mindfulness practices, including becoming more cognisant of bodily states, breathing and arousal levels, and believed we needed to work more actively with bodily awareness with very dysregulated patients. In my own work, this has often meant guiding people through body scans as well as being consistently curious about what might be going on in their bodies in specific moments.

The power of body awareness

As well as an in-depth psychoanalytic training, I earlier undertook an integrative psychotherapy training that included a substantial amount of body understanding, based on the theories of Reich (1945), Keleman (1975), Lowen (1975) and others. My training especially examined how defences get structured in the body. In recent years, I have been trying to bring these understandings into my psychotherapy practice and supervision. I set up a workshop in the Tavistock for therapists and trainees to think about trauma, neuroscience and the body, aiming to enhance awareness of embodiment, including of the embodied counter-transference. I also, like others (Sletvold, 2014), ask supervisees to include their somatic countertransference in session notes and I do more live supervision, including physically role-playing patients. This was because I too often heard case descriptions that conveyed little sense of embodied states, voice tone or gestural feel, without which I struggled to make sense of sessions. Increasing awareness of body states, their own and clients', has had a powerful effect on supervisees work.

For example, one trainee psychotherapist, who I call Mark, had been seeing Bryn, an 8-year-old boy, three times weekly for over two years, and receiving weekly individual supervision on the case. Bryn was born a twin. Both were healthy at birth, although their mother suffered with post-natal depression. She always favoured Bryn's twin and at 18 months in a tragic incident this favourite twin got his neck tangled in the curtain cord and died by hanging. Bryn was present. Mother then entered a deep depression, becoming unable to care for Bryn or his older sister. They moved in with the maternal grandmother, returning some six months later to the home where the tragedy occurred.

In therapy Bryn was a challenge to work with, resorting constantly to manic, aggressive actions, very active, barely able to contact feelings. He constantly blocked attempts by Mark to think with him, generally presenting as omnipotent, defiant, self-critical, and destructive. Mark's account of presenting in the workshop now follows.

When invited to get up and embody Bryn in front of the group I initially felt my body tense and heart race. Graham encouraged me to find a place in the middle of the group, where he had placed some chairs. I stood, hoping to settle. A shift occurred: I felt myself drawn to Graham's words, encouraging me to become Bryn and talk as him in the first person. An instinct told me I needed to be on the floor, I took a deep breath and once there, began to feel anxious again: where do I start?

My attempts to recall a specific scene triggered anxious energy in my abdomen and chest. I felt that I couldn't move. I heard Graham ask me to describe what was going on inside.

I struggled initially, and then a shift occurred. No longer occupied with thoughts, I began to feel heavy, as if weighted into the floor, even imagining that I would be pulled right into it. Graham asked what I was feeling. I said that I felt heavy and weighed down (in body and mind). Graham asked what was happening in the different areas of my body. Attention was drawn to my right leg and I noticed that it was shaking, going into spasm. A powerful feeling of being stuck was prominent. I noticed myself leaning to the side as if I might topple over. Something was happening that I had little control over, but I stayed with this, sensing its significance.

I found it difficult to verbalise my experience. I heard Graham say that he felt a tremendous sadness. With Graham naming the sadness, I too felt a wash of grief and my eyes filled, tears falling down my right cheek, into my hair and ear. I cannot recall what happened next. I think Graham named depression. This resonated strongly. Without the usual defences of mania, grievances or self-abasement, I could feel first hand some of the strength of Bryn's powerful depression. Afterwards the group and myself processed the experience. The palpable sadness resonated and I continued to feel heavy, and later, very tired.

Mark saw Bryn five days later due to his mum cancelling the next planned session. The experience stayed with Mark throughout the weekend. Before the meeting with Bryn he met with the mother, and a new space opened to talk about Bryn's deceased twin. Unusually, mum could think about Bryn's experience, not her own, of this loss.

Bryn's next session was atypical. Mark reported looking forward to it rather than his normal tense bracing. Bryn seemed more contented, reporting receiving three smiley faces at school. He then talked about being at his dad's house, expressing anger and despair about his dad moving house again, insisting that he really didn't want his dad to move because he is feeling settled now. Bryn then said that it was the second anniversary of his dad's dog's death. He was sitting on the sofa, and his head dropped and he began to sob. Without it yet being named, although this happened later, clearly both were in touch with the tragic loss of Bryn's twin. He continued to sob for much of the session, coming close to Mark. Between sobs, he asked Mark many questions, such as 'Have you ever had to move from a house you don't want to?' Have you ever lost a dog? He desperately needed someone to understand his experience, of loss and pain. When Mark talked about this Bryn showed clear relief. Both moved between relief, laughter, tears. Mark, more present to his own emotions than usual, said how connected they felt to each other, and he felt very paternal.

Previously Bryn had almost never been able to stay with any upset. Usually his despair and sadness shifted quickly to mania, attacking and omnipotent states. This sadness was a new experience for both, one that could now be built upon. It was triggered by Bryn's therapist having a new experience of being in touch with Bryn's deep emotional states via his own embodied awareness.

Summary

This chapter has stressed the importance of working at a body-aware level. Damasio (2012) helpfully showed how emotions are bodily processes, our brains constantly picking up cues from the external environment (e.g. threats) and the internal environment (e.g. heart racing). Damasio (2012) describes how our brains constantly monitor body states, regulating internal milieu to maintain homeostasis. Interoception, our awareness of our body states, can be central to good therapeutic outcomes and interestingly is also a key outcome in long-term meditation (Farb *et al.*, 2015).

As Damasio (2012) says, consciousness emerges when 'self comes to mind', including becoming aware of bodily signals to ourselves. In other words, emotional regulation develops initially from cortical 'top-down' regulation, deliberate conscious attention, but eventually becomes more bottom-up emotional regulation, which is non-conscious, procedural and second nature (Chiesa *et al.*, 2013).

Helping someone to bear and regulate their emotions is often a precursor of self-reflection, whereas being emotionally overwhelmed triggers subcortical limbic system activity that interferes with self-reflective brain circuitry. People like Paula, Myra, Bryn and Mick are often out of touch with their bodily states and rely either on precocious mental development (Winnicott, 1953) or muscular second-skin body busyness (Bick, 1968) to hold themselves together. I have emphasised how increased body awareness can lead to shifts towards quieter, less verbal states in which deep relaxation and just 'going-on-being' can occur.

This sense of oneself as embodied is, Damasio (1999) thinks, the root of feelings of having a sense of self. He rather beautifully denotes this conscious sense of oneself as 'stepping into the light', which he describes as 'a powerful metaphor for consciousness, for the birth of the knowing mind, for the simple and yet momentous coming of the sense of self into the world of the mental' (p. 3). Paula described something like this, a kind of eureka moment, when she became aware of what her body was doing, stating how in such moments her sense of herself was experienced anew. Many report something similar in mindfulness, which encourages a gently curious awareness of responses to external and internal stimuli. This is something that traumatised people often struggle to manage. Such nurturing of conscious self-awareness, including of body states, has an important place in how we practice psychotherapy with traumatised patients, as I describe in the next chapter.

Chapter 9

Trauma and treading carefully

Learning from mistakes: Rory

For many years I fell into classic errors when working with trauma, especially early developmental trauma, mistakes that had understandable roots, both personally and professionally. In recent years we have re-thought trauma and developed new clinical approaches.

I saw a young man who I call Rory in a GP practice many decades ago. While riding his bicycle he was thrown to the ground and mugged violently by local youth. On meeting he seemed friendly, appropriately nervous but rather cut-off and edgy. I had expected that he, like most, would be glad of the opportunity to talk, that processing the incident would bring relief. In fact, the opposite transpired. He quickly became agitated, moving his body jerkily, as if having tics, his eyes faraway. I found myself holding my breath anxiously, and I felt cold, my mind seemingly shutting down, something I have often experienced with traumatised patients.

The more I enquired, the more his agitation increased. I intuitively changed tack, instead asking how he was feeling in the room with me. He struggled but with careful questioning I discovered that in response to my earlier questions he had begun to experience flashbacks, which he admitted he was often assailed by. His flashbacks left him feeling unsafe about even leaving his flat. He had not been to work for several weeks.

I was naïve about trauma at the time, knowing little about flashbacks, dissociation or states such as depersonalisation or derealisation. In truth I was out of my depth. I don't hold myself too responsible. At that time people knew little about the effects of trauma on the brain and body. Thankfully I had some training in understanding somatic states and asked Rory about his bodily feelings, such as his clenched hands, and his breathing (which was shallow and fast). He could speak more easily about his bodily sensations than the trauma, and calmed somewhat. I found myself managing my own breathing, which had become tight and shallow, while asking him about his. He seemed more at ease by the end of the session and agreed to return next week. I had got lucky in asking about body states, using skills learnt in other contexts, but I lacked the knowledge to really help him.

In supervision my advice was mainly to go slowly, but that he won't get better until he could process the trauma. Thus, the next week I carried on as before. Again, he retreated into what I now know to be dissociated states. I knew something was wrong. I felt I was failing him, that his mental state was getting worse, but I lacked the understanding to work with this. When Rory did not return, I called him, and he said that he felt worse after the session and thought it best to stop for now. I felt awful, but I now think he did what was right for him. The last thing he needed was to have his trauma re-triggered by prematurely talking about it. I discussed the case with the referring GP, a psychiatric nurse visited him and he was placed on anti-anxiety medication. I do not know what happened after that. I was left with many questions about what constitutes good therapeutic work after trauma.

A personal aside

Like many in the helping professions, I honed my skills in understanding distress in the cauldron of a dysfunctional family in which adults relied on children to help manage their own feelings. I learnt early to be hyperresponsive to mood changes, and how to make others feel better. For better or worse I was good at this, learning that being attentive to others' distress often calmed them down. Such skills reaped rewards in a family where conflict could quickly escalate, but we need more than this to work with trauma.

When I eventually found psychotherapy, I realised that much of the role was helping people's distress in similar ways to those learnt in my family, and something clicked. In my own therapies, I experienced relief when my feelings were heard, and I was helped to bear distressing early life events that I had brushed aside, some genuinely traumatic. Life felt richer as I became braver about bearing and staying with difficulty. Not surprisingly I became a passionate advocate of therapy.

When I started working therapeutically I built on these lessons. Both humanistic and psychoanalytic therapy taught the importance of painful feelings being heard, borne and expressed, the relief this can give and the risks of leaving such experiences buried. On becoming a therapist, I felt relatively at ease helping others manage painful experiences, and working through such issues in the transference. Despite long, often painstaking work, I saw dramatic life changes and people becoming more easeful and self-accepting. Yet there were some for whom this did not seem to work, like Rory, and Fred discussed below. With them patterns emerged that left me feeling out of my depth.

Fred

Fred, 10 years old, was in foster care, after having been physically abused by his stepfather. He had been locked in his room without food or a toilet, and subjected to blistering verbal assaults. He had for the last year been settling well with a thoughtful foster carer. He was referred after hurting a child and threatening another at school. In initial meetings I was struck by Fred's ability to describe what had happened. When we eventually started psychotherapy, I was surprised that he could play symbolically and he could play out fictional and real-life events.

In one session he enacted a scene in which he, scared, called the police. Holding a pretend phone, I said, 'Hello, Police here, how can I help?' He replied, 'My stepdad is hurting me.' I say, 'Oh dear, that sounds terrible, what is he doing?' Fred described being scared to leave his room in case he was hurt, but hating staying there as his mum was being hurt. I said, 'Oh dear, that sounds so frightening, horrible, that should not happen to any boy of your age. What would you like me to do?' Fred looked uncertain. I asked whether I should come and arrest his stepfather, and he said yes. Then he said he must stop the call as his stepfather was outside the room.

Such work left me hopeful. He seemed able to communicate memories of traumatic experiences in symbolic form through play, allowing us to process them together. To an extent this was true, and he seemed calmer in the following weeks. The play then took a different turn. He enacted scenes of his stepfather being angry and violent. I joined in, assuming this also was a hopeful development, good therapeutic work helping to process his experiences. The scenes were physically and verbally aggressive.

Unbeknown to me, this play was having a bad effect. Fred became agitated at home, and there were incidents at school, the first for months. His sleep had worsened and he was having nightmares. Most worrying, he told his foster carer that he had been seeing his stepfather's face, and evidently had been having flashbacks.

I realised belatedly that the dramatic re-enactments had re-evoked his trauma, leaving him fragile. I needed to review my approach. While traumatic experiences are too often brushed under the carpet when they need to be dealt with, here the timing and approach were unhelpful, and indeed re-traumatising. I changed tack, not encouraging memories, allowing more space for the ordinary play that boys indulge in at Fred's age. This seemed less like 'real therapy' to me. We played emotionally neutral games, football, building towers, duller activities. He now could settle down, be like other boys, experience the safe uneventfulness of ordinary life, build up trust in the predictability of his new life, a needed contrast to the chaotic terror he grew up with.

Middle childhood years are often marked by calmer, ordinary game-playing, and social learning. Psychoanalysis describes this as the latency period, when powerful urges, sexual and otherwise, dampen down, at least until adolescence. In my day, this was marked by collecting stamps or cards, or playing with toy cars or conkers. Latency is known for less emotional lability, although not for dysregulated children who have suffered maltreatment like Fred.

Fred needed an experience of safety, an absence of threat, even if this makes for uneventful therapy with too much football! Even football and ball-throwing help embed social skills, turn-taking and trust, all vitally important for such children. Fred needed this before re-encountering his traumatic past. It is easier to face and process difficult experiences when one has developed some sense of calm and ease.

Safety first

For good reasons, therapeutic trainings encourage processing of difficult and frightening experiences, painful emotions, aggressive or despairing parts of the personality. New understandings of trauma explain why it can be vital to also build positive, safety-based feeling states.

Highly traumatised patients like Rory and Fred need preparation before approaching the extreme suffering they have endured. Putting them in touch with the trauma too quickly can be like prodding an open wound with a sharp instrument. It can trigger re-traumatisation, redoubling defences and, more worryingly, the kind of dissociative states seen in Rory and Fred.

Trauma, by definition, is overwhelming. Flashbacks feel as if terrifying past events are happening in the present, the sufferer lacking a vantage point from which to make sense of the experiences. Parts of the personality capable of providing a sense of safety, calm and trust need to be built first, a secure vantage point, from which to revisit and process difficult experiences.

It is no coincidence that many newer forms of trauma therapy, such as compassion-focused therapy (CFT) (Gilbert, 2014) or eye-movement desensitisation and reprocessing therapy (EMDR) (Parnell et al., 2013), expend much effort building up what they call resources, inner states that feel safe, easeful and self-caring. CFT facilitates clients to stimulate healthy branches of the parasympathetic nervous system by, for example, a breathing technique called soothing-rhythmic breathing, or by imagining a safe place or a compassionate figure. EMDR practitioners similarly help traumatised people to 'install' good resources, such as a safe place or a wise or nurturing figure that become internal *imagos* to rely on.

Such active techniques are not for everyone, but they certainly take seriously the dangers of re-traumatisation. Installing good resources is rather like what psychoanalysis describes as installing a good internal object, something that too often was thought to happen almost automatically. Therapeutic technique often rightly focuses on taking up what we call the negative transference. Yet many of the most disturbed children and adults need good experiences and reliable figures, inside or outside the self, including their therapist, to enable sufficient trust, before the negative can be successfully borne.

Our first reactions, when fearful or in danger, is for our sympathetic nervous system to fire up, giving rise to tense bodies, shallow breathing, faster heart rates, knotted stomachs and a range of psychological processes such as fight and flight. While danger, real or imaginary, looms, reflective, thoughtful or empathic circuitry is tuned right down. After serious trauma, dissociative numbed states are also often triggered, particularly following ongoing multiple traumas. The dangers increase when there have been too few good experiences to provide emotional inoculation against the effects of bad experiences.

Many children live in a world of danger, threat or even terror, even in contexts such as classrooms where other children are interpreting the same environment as ordinarily benign. Such children need help building up a 'window of tolerance' (see Figure 9.1), which provides a safe place to return to, a vantage point from which to visit more difficult experiences.

Less serious cases

The importance of working with positive affect states also applies to less traumatised cases, where sometimes staying with difficulty is also not enough. Isobel, 17 years old, had received some genuine affection and care in her family, but had had an absent, reactive father and a mother prone to manage her anxiety with a false breeziness and positivity. Isobel

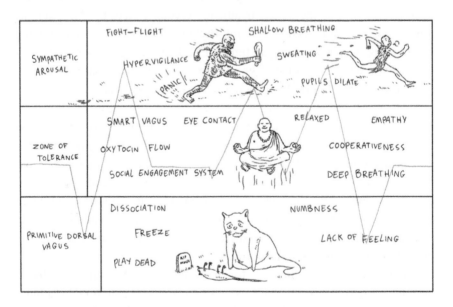

Figure 9.1 Autonomic nervous systems.
Based on Porges (2011) and Ogden (2006).

was depressed and anxious. Several years of therapy were spent working through her despair. Isobel could now almost consider previously feared negative emotional states as rather like old friends about whom she had mixed feelings, but with whom she could now get along. This was real progress, but she still felt unable to enjoy many areas of life.

She was frightened of dark, enclosed spaces and for example could not travel on the London underground system. We processed how she was punished as a young child by being sent into a cupboard by an abusive nanny, leaving her feeling terrified. The nanny was subsequently dismissed. She also remembered getting lost in some woods and being terrified, fearing she might die. We made links with her past experiences and looked at the symbolic meaning, the fear in the family of dark psychic states, her mother's terror of suffocating in gloom and depression, the fear of underground, unconscious feelings. All this was true but only got us so far. Unlike serious cases of developmental trauma, Isobel's trauma was specific, and in the context of a life in which she felt genuinely loved and cared for. Nonetheless her traumas needed addressing.

From therapy, she began to feel less plagued by anxiety. However, she was as fearful as ever of dark spaces. She had a nagging sense of failure, symbolic of several areas of her life where she felt inhibited and stymied and, to use her words, 'psychologically frozen'.

My work shifted at this point. I realised I needed to help her re-experience childhood feelings of terror, really get to know the states of mind and body she went into. Before this, I helped her to remember good experiences when she had felt safe and loved. We actively returned to these when the fear became too much. Having established a sense of safety to come back to, we worked on learning to get to know and bear the difficult feelings in her body. We found ways in which she could look after those feelings so they did not continue controlling her life. This was in part desensitisation, as behavioural therapists do, acclimatising her to what she had been so fearful of. Moving backwards and forwards to the good experiences, and the accompanying bodily sensations of safety, allowed her to venture out into the more terrifying ones.

Of course, at some point she needed to take the plunge into darkness. My psychoanalytic training had not equipped me to facilitate positive behavioural change. I even questioned whether it was my job to help her do this. In the event I did, but often by using convoluted pseudo-interpretations to mask what were really encouragements. I said things like 'it is hard for you to believe that I think you really could do this' or 'maybe you are clinging to an idea that you are still 5 years old and the darkness will feel as frightening'. Thankfully she knew what I was up to, at one point asking wryly, 'Are you actually encouraging me?'

She eventually, literally a step at a time, ventured into places that frightened her. For example, she risked going down steps in the tube system, gradually increasing the depth, while she monitored her breathing and other signs of stress. She also began to feel more confident in other areas, taking risks at work and in relationships, developing more belief in her capacities. I worried that I was encouraging pseudo-capacities, masking or glossing over her difficulties. I feared that if I became a too positive figure, I might become unable to pick up any negative transference, such as how I might represent untrustworthy parental figures. However, we need to help people feel good, in addition to managing unhappiness, otherwise we are only doing half the job of therapy.

A famous early example of a psychoanalyst working this way was Michael Balint (1968). In his book *The Basic Fault* he described a patient with lots of potential who always let herself down. She was bright but failed her exams, lively and sociable but could not manage relationships. She had learnt to keep her feet firmly planted on the ground and said to Balint that, despite wishing to, she had never managed to do a somersault. His famous, non-interpretative response was 'What about it now?' At this point she got up and somersaulted across the room. Balint described this as a turning point, a 'new beginning', after which 'many changes followed in her emotional, social, and professional life, all towards greater freedom and elasticity' (p. 129). Balint was not an overly positive therapist, and did not shirk pain and difficulty, neither should we. However, we need to get the right balance between focusing on good and difficult experiences.

Allan

Like Isobel, Allan, 15, did not suffer the kind of trauma that gives rise to dissociative states. However, he was crippled by anxiety. His mother was depressed when he was born, and prone to fits of rage. His parents' shaky marriage did not survive his third year. He never knew when his mother would take to her bed, have a meltdown, or occasionally, be in a happy mood. The latter was more manic excitement, her seemingly positive states always teetering on the edge of disaster. She often railed at him, blaming him when she was upset, reacting disproportionately to minor misdemeanours such as an untidy room or spilt food. He was extremely anxious and self-blaming, and with me was inordinately polite and careful.

If something upset him, such as someone being critical, it unleashed waves of self-loathing. His self-hatred was exacerbated by shame about his sexuality, as a young gay adolescent. He believed that whatever went wrong was his fault, that he was deeply flawed. His self-hatred, once unleashed, ran rampant, leaving him with no still, safe place inside. Not surprisingly, he resorted to self-harm when the self-loathing became too much, and he had overdosed a few times.

Young people like Allan quickly get triggered into despairing states and, like many trauma patients, often have few good internal resources to rely on. With them working too directly too soon with pain and despair can feel like there is no escape from that deep dark ditch. We should not facilitate a false manic positivity but we do need to help people find a safe enough place from where to start processing difficult experiences. In the middle of pain, terror, despair or anxiety, people need to trust that there is something better as well.

We need to create an emotionally and bodily attuned viewing point from which to observe and process difficult experiences. This is what a good mother does for a young child, lending them her prefrontal cortex, conveying her own understanding that the current experience is bearable, understandable and indeed, will pass. Mindfulness teaches this too, that all experiences pass, but also that we can cultivate a place from which to bear the complexity and difficulty of the present moment.

Allan's was not a classic case of trauma, but much of his life was lived in the storms of his mother's moods, and he had become a cipher for her feeling states. When young, he took on her worldview, including that when things went wrong someone should be blamed, generally him, leading to shame and self-attack. Yet the alacrity with which he developed a safer viewing point suggested that he had also had good experiences, presumably from other adults in his life, such as his grandmother, whose mention always led to a softening in him.

One week, quite early in his therapy, he came full of angst. He had been playing football and had got into a spat with another boy who had screamed at him for not passing the ball quickly enough. Among other insults, he was told that he was letting the team down. He was distraught, filled with self-hatred and hopelessness. Initially I needed to just stay with his feelings, showing empathy, that I understood something of his state of mind, enquiring about his immediate reactions. He said, 'I just feel shit, I am shit, this is my life, I fucking hate it, hate myself. I just want to die.'

Next though I asked about this boy, what he was like, and questioned with some curiosity what might have been going on for him. This was a new idea. Like many vigilant children, he could read other minds better than most, after all, his passport to safety was working out his mother's moods. However, he had never learnt to be genuinely interested in what another might be thinking or feeling. His mentalising had been defensive, he was able to vigilantly read another's feelings, but not easily 'feel with them', nor see things from their point of view.

It transpired that the aggressive boy was a volatile young man with a violent father, also a bully. I wondered aloud, as curiously as I could, whether the problem might lay in the other boy, not Allan, that perhaps the boy had 'issues' of his own. I said, 'So isn't it possible that he acted inappropriately, that he was out of order?' There was a deeper breath than usual, a sense of relief, a surprise that it might not all be his fault.

In ensuing sessions, we thought more about this other boy. He too it seems was troubled by his sexuality and had previously made a sexual advance to Allan. He had suffered bullying from his father, and was now making others feel bad in the way he had been made to feel. Allan had a perfect 'valency' to receive such treatment, given his past. I began to question how Allan felt when treated like this. 'Was this fair? Did he "deserve" to be treated so badly?' The idea that he might be entitled to decent treatment, that he should receive ordinary respect, seemed new. As a young child he had had no choice but to believe his mother's words, to assume that when she was upset it was his fault. When young he could not afford to reject his mother, so he took the blame on himself, all too common in young children.

In time, we could think about his relationship with his mother. When her mood states flooded him, we could examine their effect on his body and emotions. He learnt to watch himself feeling responsible for her feelings, and learnt to disengage a bit from this.

The psychoanalyst Ronald Fairbairn long ago (1962) described this dynamic with the metaphor that, for a child, 'it is better to be a sinner in a world ruled by God than to live in a world ruled by the devil' (pp. 66–67). In a young, traumatised psyche a split often occurs, badness being internalised while goodness is projected out. Allan was a master of this and the idea that it could be another way around was novel but hope-inducing. He began to realise that he need not feel so responsible for his mother's unhappiness, just as he need not be blamed, or feel self-blaming, for what happened on the football pitch. He became more able to think about other people's motivations, thoughts and agendas, including his mother's, and the other boy's.

He felt huge relief as he began to realise that other people's feelings were not necessarily his problem. This shifted how he felt in other relationships. He told me,

> It is funny, I used to feel that everyone had to like me, or else it was a disaster. But last week when B disapproved, I just felt, well, maybe that's his issue, not mine, if he does not like me for it, I can manage, it's not the end of the world. I don't need to collect friends now, I can build friendships that are good for me, and turn down others.

Over time this all bore fruit. Throughout his two-year therapy the theme of 'it might not be my fault' threaded through as a central motif. As he began to experiment with dating, his most needy feelings quickly surfaced, and we had to face his lack of confidence, about whether he could be attractive, acceptable and most of all, loveable. In intimacy, old patterns become powerfully re-enacted and therapy is the perfect place to work these through. He learnt to trust that other people's moods were just that, *their* moods, and he did not have to solve their issues.

When he was turned down by a boy he had asked out, he was at first aghast, on the brink of self-harming again. However, as I encouraged him to try to make sense of what might be going on for this boy, he felt better. On another occasion, he was on the receiving end of a coruscating telling off from a teacher who he was afraid of, but whose approval he sought. Mortified, he initially retreated in a hang-dog way. However, now he was able to protest about the inappropriateness of how he was treated. Other people were becoming more real, with their own thoughts, feelings and histories, and he could be interested in them, less worried about pleasing them. This all depended on cultivating some sense of inner safety, a feeling that he was all right in himself. This in turn was helped by making sense of his history, especially how he had become so over-responsive and self-blaming. His earlier once adaptive patterns had caused him trouble, but he was realising that they need not be a life sentence.

Jade: a case of abuse

By the time I saw 14-year-old Jade, some years later, my understanding of trauma had thankfully increased. Jade had been sexually abused over years by her maternal uncle. Her mother too had been abused, an intergenerational pattern. Jade struggled with friendships, often felt rejected and a victim. She was placed with her aunt, her father's sister, by social services. The aunt and uncle had raised biological children, had been carefully assessed and she had her first experience of a safe protective home. She had a good relationship with her father who remained a positive presence, albeit not deemed competent to look after her.

I had learnt by now that Jade, like most trauma survivors, would not be able to address traumatic incidents too quickly. The complexity of my task was increased by being a male therapist. I learnt from school how she could frequently withdraw into dissociative 'fugue-like' states, and was easily triggered into flashbacks.

I immediately made it clear that we could go slowly, not talk about anything too difficult until she was ready. When I said this she visibly relaxed. Much of the initial work concerned very ordinary issues, what happened in her friendships, how she was getting on in drama club, her struggles with adapting to a big new school. On the surface, this might not have looked like psychotherapy but I have learnt that building up trust in ordinary good experiences is crucial. I made sure that we gave plenty of space for things she was beginning to feel good about, especially feelings of being cherished by her aunt. I would explore these positive feelings in detail, asking exactly how she felt, what was going on in her body, what the warm feelings were like.

One week she told me about having a birthday sleepover with close girlfriends. She had a smile on her face and was clearly unused to such happy feelings. I said, 'How great it is that you have had such a good time, that you have people around who care about you and can look after you, who keep you safe.' She smiled, looking almost tearful. I asked what it was like to have her friends over, what were the best things about the experience? A few years back I would have felt that asking about 'the best things' was defensive, manically avoiding the painful ones, but by now I knew that Jade needed such hopeful parts of herself building. She told me about the fun, the giggling, the lack of worry. The best part, she said, was the look of love on her aunt's face. I said, 'What does it feel like when you imagine her face like that?' She smiled, her eyes moistening, saying, 'I don't know how to describe it, sort of warm, soft, a bit dreamy.' I asked her to really hold on to that feeling as one to go back to, checking where she felt it, what was happening in her chest, face, muscles. I was hoping that such good feelings would become a body memory.

Over time we built up a repertoire of such good feelings. We talked about her bedroom becoming a safe place where she could relax and feel at ease. She said, 'And when I am there my breathing, it sort of, becomes soft, gentle. Sometimes, it sounds daft, but I almost purr, I just know

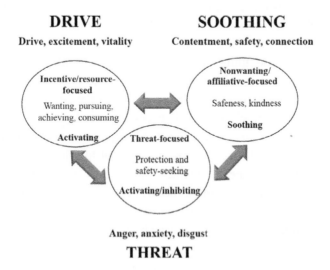

Figure 9.2 Three-circles model.

nothing bad will happen there.' We spent time getting to know this kind of breathing, comparing it to her breathing when anxious, becoming familiar with the journey backwards and forwards from her threat system to her soothing, calming affiliative systems, as described in the three-circle model (see Figure 9.2) (Gilbert, 2014). In trauma, we try to build up the system represented by the soothing, calming system, where we can feel love, compassion, self-care and relaxed well-being. Jade was building trust in her own lovability, through her new family, therapy and friends. Her window of tolerance, and her soothing system, were becoming places that could be trusted and returned to in times of stress.

Occasionally, like at exam time, her anxiety skyrocketed. I said, 'You sound like you feel like the hugest disaster is about to happen, It really feels like that. What is happening now in your body, your breathing?' 'Yes,' she said, almost surprised, 'I am tight, tense, hardly breathing.' At this she relaxed, deliberately breathing more deeply, and in almost the next sentence said, 'Actually, I know my aunt won't care how I do as long as I do my best, that's what counts.'

Not surprisingly, when she was approached by a boy who liked her, and who she also quite liked, her stress went through the roof. She started having nightmares and occasional flashbacks returned. She was scared by her feelings of attraction, and memories of her abuse flashed back. Not surprisingly, some of her experiences with her abusive uncle had been pleasurable, including sexually, as she guiltily admitted to me.

'That is all so confusing', I said with feeling, trying to normalise that she felt some good things in the abuse, the specialness, even sexual pleasure, while I also stressed how inappropriate and wrong his actions were. She was struggling to separate out feelings about her uncle and the boy, but slowly some clear space between them emerged. Jade had never trusted that it was safe to be excited, have pleasure and seek out good things. Her drive and pleasure systems had felt too threatening and been almost turned off. For her, excitement and anxiety were almost the same, and of course they use similar bodily systems. Slowly she learnt to separate out feelings like anxiety, excitement and fear. Jade began to experience ordinary teenage sexual feelings with anxious pleasure rather than terror or dread.

For a long time, she was easily triggered into panic before knowing what was happening, and sometimes even dissociated. In time, she got to know the triggers, the first signs, such as her heart beating faster, muscles tensing, breathing getting shallower. We could track this in sessions. 'Hmmm', I might say, looking at her arms and mimicking her, tensing myself, holding tight and breathing shallowly. She laughed and her body softened. We practised this in sessions, acting tense and seeing what happened, examining what happened in her body as she became fearful, both in role play and by thinking about her bodily responses to actual anxiety provoking situations. She learnt that she could take a deep breath and regulate herself. We returned often to the experiences of safeness that we had built up, that could now be more trusted.

We had built bridges so she could more easily return to her window of tolerance, not flip into hyperanxiety or numbed states. Indeed, her window of tolerance was broadening, and pathways back to it were getting easier to find. This allowed Jade to try out her drive and play systems more too, and she began to enjoy new activities, like a dance class, a singing group and performing.

As safeness developed we could begin to confront some of the trauma, a little at a time. If she edged towards dissociative states we would focus on basic body sensations, like feeling her feet on the ground, or the tingling in her fingers. My aim was re-embodying and staying present, bearing whatever arose, but from our newly developed viewing point, a constant to-ing and fro-ing from safety and out of it, learning that she could return to her window of tolerance, recognising when she was moving out of it.

When we are triggered into sympathetic nervous system reactivity prefrontal parts of our brains turn off and survival is all that counts. This is even more the case in dorsal vagal-led numbed dissociative states. As Bessel van der Kolk (2014), showed, parts of the brain central to language, such as Broca's region, become inactive in such frozen states. In *Macbeth*, Shakespeare exhorted that we 'give sorrow words, the grief that does not speak knits up the o'er wrought heart and bids it break' (Act IV, Scene III). However, this is not possible until we feel sufficiently safe. By helping patients like Jade move into their window of tolerance, difficult experiences can be processed without re-triggering trauma.

Such work takes patience, many steps backwards as well as forwards. By the end of our sessions together, Jade could talk about her trauma with me and others close to her. She started to feel that she was a whole person, with capacities and a future, not just a traumatised person, the 'damaged goods' she had once felt herself to be. She now had robust hopeful aspects of her personality that were solidly there to rely on.

A healthy life depends on being able to embrace good experiences as well as managing difficult ones. In psychotherapy we can focus too much, and too soon, on negative emotions, defence mechanisms, trauma. However, we also need to develop our two primary positive emotional systems.

One is the soothing system, linked to affiliation, attachment and feeling secure in relationships. This is where we experience safety and well-being, so badly needed by trauma survivors, like Jade, Rory and Allan. The other main positive affect system is the appetitive or seeking (Panksepp and Biven, 2012) system, which leads to pleasure, hope and excitement and is linked with moving towards and not away from experiences, to increasing good feelings, not just avoiding negative ones. Jade by the end could inhabit both positive systems without feeling overwhelmed. Traumatised patients need help to trust in a soothing, safeness system, a prerequisite for both the pleasures of the seeking system and the ability to manage difficult experiences. Focusing prematurely on the trauma can backfire, as I and my early patients painfully learnt.

Chapter 10

Angels and devils

Sadism and violence in children

Sadism, aggression and addiction

It can be uncomfortable to think of children having violent or sadistic personality traits. As Anne Alvarez (1995) makes clear, 'staring evil in the eye', without shirking painful truths, requires courage. Some see children as 'angels' with positive natures, naïvely believing that kindness and love always shine through, turning a blind eye to disturbing realities. Others see some children as innately destructive, even potentially evil. We must steer a course between the Scylla and Charybdis of these views.

Mary Bell was an extreme infamous example. Before her eleventh birthday she had murdered several children, including strangling a 3-year-old in local wasteland. Chillingly she returned to carve an 'M' into his stomach, cut his hair off and mutilate his penis. Mary was also a victim, her mother was a prostitute who offered her to men for sex. Mary 'accidentally' fell out of windows, and her mother gave her sleeping pills that she said were sweets. Yet judge and jury understandably saw her as a callous psychopath, a massive danger to children. As professionals, we need to understand both the abusing and abused aspects of the personality, both victim and perpetrator in the same person, and try to get inside their minds, which is no easy task.

Our first job is to take in awful realities and manage our own horror. Take Jamie Bulger, murdered by 10-year-olds Jon Venables and Robert Thompson. Bulger had paint thrown in his eyes, was stamped on, beaten with bricks and an iron bar, batteries reportedly pushed into his anus, 10 skull fractures and 43 major injuries. It is hard to feel anything but revulsion and antipathy for the perpetrators, but we know they too were victims (c.f. Morrison, 2011).

Many cases I see are hot potatoes, referred because of high anxiety in professional systems, especially if there is violence, or sexual acting out. Typically, 8-year-old Bill had been caught in sexual play in toilets with younger children. Some saw him as already a callous serial sex offender who should be excluded from school permanently. Others were fond of him, seeing him as an innocent victim. He was living with his aunt. His mother was a drug user who prostituted herself and his father was her pimp. He often came to school unkempt and dirty. His appearance, academic work and social skills had improved since living with his aunt.

Bill's case raises typical dilemmas. He could be aggressive and cruel, had few friends and enjoyed hurting other children, although this had abated in recent months. Was his cruelty a way of projecting feelings into others that he could not bear in himself? Was the lessening aggression a sign of feeling safer, after better care from his aunt? Or was he just becoming more sophisticated in his manipulations? Was his aggression mainly cold and calculated or more reactive to frustration? Should the positive feelings he evoked in adults be trusted? He enjoyed the attention of his young female teaching assistant and often snuggled into her. Was he genuinely craving affection or was this sexualised contact masquerading as innocent affection-seeking? Such questions are typical of what needs unpicking in such cases.

Many children we work with show pleasurable sexual excitement in inflicting pain. Much compulsive addictive behaviour starts for defensive reasons, maybe as attempts to manage trauma, but can become addictive. Typically, many soldiers in war-torn areas show appetitive violence (Weierstall et al., 2013), the excitement of killing. Some child soldiers in the Congo returned to war zones to re-experience this, the return to fighting actually warding off post-traumatic stress symptoms (Weierstall et al., 2012). Aggressive and sadistic acts can be used to manage unbearable emotions, an addictive form of anti-depressant.

Similarly, in compulsive sexual behaviours brain pathways central to addiction are triggered (Voon and Potenza, 2015), particularly circuitry central to the dopaminergic system, such as the nucleus accumbens and ventral striatum (Kalivas and Volkow, 2014). People often turn towards sexually compulsive behaviour as an antidote to unmanageable feelings, just as they turn to any addiction, whether cocaine, alcohol or gambling, especially when they feel down, angry or humiliated.

The pleasure in another's suffering is probably a distortion of ordinary *schadenfreude*, in which empathic brain circuitry and fellow-feeling gets turned off (Bhanji and Delgado, 2014) and reward circuitry turned on (Jankowski and Takahashi, 2014). Linked to poorly developed emotional worlds, such perpetrators often experience a form of psychic deadness (Gilligan, 2009). Lacking the ability to bear and process emotional challenges, they often re-offend at times of stress or pain, seeking immediate relief from unbearable emotions. As my colleague Ariel Nathanson (2016) has written, many patients press what he calls their 'fuck-it button', giving rise to a triumphant thrill that overrides negative emotions.

Les, 11 years old, was caught forcing his 9-year-old brother to suck his penis. There was intergenerational sexual abuse and domestic violence, with family relationships based on fear, control and power. On our advice, Les was taken into a residential unit where he continued to be a risk to other children, more so when difficult feelings were stirred up, such as his key worker being away. Les had poor emotional vocabulary, little trust in adults and treated most people with contempt. We learnt of terrible violence towards his mother from her partners, but also acts perpetrated by Les himself, including molesting a younger child. Les seemed uncontrollably driven to act this way, more so when he was struggling emotionally. I was struck by the paucity of his empty and flat mind. His recourse to sexual stimulation, often at others' expense, was a way of feeling less dead. Until healthier ways of feeling emotionally alive developed, this would continue.

Like Les, many perpetrators have been victims of sexual offences themselves (Ogloff *et al.*, 2012) and come from backgrounds high in conflict, cruelty, neglect and a lack of nurturing, emotional care (Riser *et al.*, 2013). They often view the world, and other people, as fundamentally untrustworthy and dangerous.

In adolescence, when the dopamine system is fast developing, risks of addictive behaviours are heightened, whether to drugs, computer games, sexual and other forms of sadism. Often what starts as an understandable defence, such as hurting another to evacuate feelings of being hurt oneself, transforms into addictively pleasurable aggression. Part of our task is to work out when to work with what is below the surface, the emotional pain, and when to work overtly with the 'secondary defence' of the pleasure in the perpetration.

In Les' case therapy was not enough, he made only small inroads, which increased somewhat after careful work with professionals about boundary setting and the dangers he posed. Les' therapy ended prematurely, but interestingly he reappeared two years later after the system around him had become more reliable and less porous. He then started to make some genuine use of therapy, but only time will tell the extent to which his cold defences might give way to hopeful personality traits.

In what follows I introduce a few key themes, including the concept of the core complex and the difference between hot reactive as opposed to colder aggression, using a shorter, less successful case example and then a longer, more hopeful one.

Cold aggressors

Some aggressors show colder, more proactive forms of aggression, targeting others to get what they want. They might read minds well but lack fellow feeling. Proactive 'happy victimisers' (Smith *et al.*, 2010) can also respond reactively when angry, but their acts are often calculated, even enjoyed. Such 'cold' aggression is potentially in all of us, like a predator stalking its prey, a needed mammalian trait. However, in worrying cases, such cold traits are not balanced by humane, warm and caring impulses.

Unlike reactive children and adults who often cry out against unfairness, cold-hearted aggressors care little about their victims, lacking remorse. They are harder to treat, partly because they are less motivated to change, and highly driven by gains from aggression.

As Arsenio suggests (Arsenio and Gold, 2006), many from backgrounds where love, support and empathy were absent, come to see relationships as about power, control and getting what one wants. Many display anti-social tendencies and behavioural problems, and some are designated *callous-unemotional* (Viding and McCrory, 2018).

Callous-unemotional traits often show continuity from early years into adult life (Waller and Hyde, 2018). Many adult psychopaths were anti-social children, starting fires, torturing pets and showing cruelty. Callous-unemotional traits in children, alongside conduct disorders, increase the likelihood of criminality later. Interestingly the cold-heartedness is not just a metaphor. Low heart rate is predictive of traits like lying, fearlessness and behavioural problems (MacKinnon *et al.*, 2018).

They have low physiological arousal, minimal amygdala response when shown pictures of violence or horrific injuries and seem barely affected by another's pain (Lockwood *et al.*, 2013).

Mick, 12 years old, had a tough, steely side, his interactions based on what he could get, taking pleasure in others' pain. He was abandoned as a toddler in an orphanage overseas, where he was subjected to horrendous sexual abuse and violence. He was adopted by a man who groomed him for a paedophile ring, and was eventually taken into care. He was sexually predatory and a bully. Professionals did not know what to make of him. He could show cold cruelty, such as being found twisting the arm of another child, squeezing as hard as he could, showing icy remorseless pleasure.

In play, dolls were cut up, mutilated and tortured to evident enjoyment. I often felt chilled in his presence, dry mouthed, dreading seeing him. In one early session he told me, smirking gleefully, that he had deliberately kicked a child in the chest, breaking several ribs. Therapeutically it was important to show that I could tolerate the depth of his cruelty. Partly this comes from being able to tolerate our own potentially cruel traits, to own up to what any human is capable of.

Mick showed what are called 'core-complex' issues, a concept developed by Mervyn Glasser (1986), former director of the Portman clinic. The core complex has similarities to what is sometimes called the claustro-agoraphobic shuttle (Rey and Magagna, 1994). Often seen in sadistic, aggressive or sexually acting-out patients, it describes an inability to bear either closeness or separation, and consequent seesaw-ing between them. Mick was involved in sadomasochistic sexual acts with both boys and girls, in which he had to be in control. Such acts allowed some closeness, in classic core-complex style, avoiding the desolation of aloneness, but without the need for actual intimacy. He had masturbation fantasies reminiscent of his abuse, and sought out sexual contact and pornography that enacted similar sadomasochistic and fetishistic scenes.

Mick demonstrated typical core-complex fears of both abandonment and closeness. Dread of aloneness led to renewed contact but in an extremely controlling way. In core-complex presentations, vulnerability and abandonment are avoided via aggression and control, both distance and closeness being retained via sexual or violent enactments. Loving relating is disavowed, and softness and vulnerability denigrated (Rosen-feld, 1987). Beginning to bear painful feelings of contact with another often becomes the meat of therapeutic work, and did with Mick.

Alvarez (1992) suggested that, when working with autistic children, we must help grow 'non-autistic' parts of the personality. With callous-unemotional children like Mick we try to help grow non-callous traits, without being naïve or Pollyannaish.

To trigger interest in psychological states, I began playing with toy animals in front of him, talking in the character's voices. Any kindness or caring I enacted with the animals was cruelly broken up. When he eventually began to play himself, I witnessed gleefullness at violence and killing. Chilling as this was, it allowed me to talk about his feelings, acknowledging with as little judgement as I could muster, his pleasure in sadism and violence. I had to show I could bear but not collude with the horrors of his mind.

Hopeful moments in time crept in. In one session, he momentarily hesitated, and I sensed a shift, something I often would have missed. This time I asked where his mind was. He looked surprised and said, 'I was thinking about Miss X', who I knew was a kind figure from his orphanage. Such flickering self-awareness signalled a re-contacting of better experiences. I simply said, 'Wow Mick you really are having thoughts, and memories, even remembering nice things.' To my surprise, this led to him voicing a wish that he was still at his primary school, saying, 'I think about it lots of times.'

Any small progress depended on me absolutely facing his mind's horrors, but also building on real positives that emerged with our increased trust. Sometimes hope showed in simple ways. His pencil kept breaking, something that would have infuriated him some months before, but now he could say, 'Ok I can do it', as he determinedly sharpened it, building on a new belief that difficulties and ruptures could be repaired. This happened after he had attacked me vehemently, accusing me of only seeing him just for the money, and calling me a 'paedo', and a 'saddo'. He resisted hope that he might trust me, but the hope was there, a seed of belief in goodness. My steadfastness and constant presence got through to him, eventually, resulting in some softening.

In the following months he started to permit pauses, listening, thinking. He could not say what he was thinking but began to allow me to muse aloud about his thoughts, no longer pushing me away. I might say, 'Well it's not easy to trust anyone, especially that idiot saddo, Dr Music. It must have been easier when Mick didn't trust anyone, hate and anger can be much easier.' After such comments I sometimes sensed some relief where previously only cold disdain had been present.

In time, small memories crept into the room, such as of Miss X, the benign figure from the orphanage. He started to trust that I too could care, as well as his foster carer. I noticed him becoming interested in me, watching my expressions, even helping clear up a little after sessions. Similar changes were spotted at home and school.

In time he became nearer managing more feelings. He had struggled with a therapy break, during which he was unhappy and became aggressive to those around him. He could not acknowledge any dependence on me until I forcefully said, in 'therapist-centred' style, about how sad I felt that he did not believe that he was in my mind over the break. He looked slightly shaken, a tiny chink in his armour, but quickly squirmed out of this feeling. I struggled, as often, with how hopeful to be. It is easy to feel falsely hopeful with such children.

My therapy with Mick was not the most successful, in part because his foster placement broke down and he too had to leave the area. Placements of children with callous traits often fail, in part because such children are hard to like or warm to. Progress had been slow anyway, and he had continued to bully and manipulate other children, albeit slightly less. He left as some soft edges were surfacing and I will never know if these could have been built upon. I remain hopeful that they could, if slowly. Research in the Portman clinic with offenders shows that genuine personality change often occurs via psychotherapy, but the evidence suggests that such change does not show until about three years into treatment. There are no quick fixes with this patient group.

Mick, typically, was on course for a criminal record, and was already stealing, bullying, causing serious injury and damage to property. We are not sure why some children experiencing terrible neglect and abuse are more likely to develop in this way than others. Some (e.g. Viding and McCrory, 2018) suggest, on the basis of twin studies, that there are genetic influences. However, I have never come across a violent or psychopathic person who had a normal childhood, and any trip into a high-security prison reveals unthinkably horrendous stories (Gullhaugen and Nøttestad, 2012).

Negative life events such as neglect, maltreatment (Kimonis *et al.*, 2014) and low maternal warmth (Bisby *et al.*, 2017) are linked to the development of callous-unemotional traits and psychopathy. My belief is that neglect, such as an extreme absence of good experiences, and the shutdown seen in dissociative states, both often lead to such coldness. Whatever the causes, children like Mick are a huge challenge to treat.

Sophia: hot aggression with core-complex elements

Some commit impulsive 'hot-blooded' aggressive acts, rather than cold ones. They feel easily provoked and retaliate, often because something feels 'unfair'. Such reactivity can be fuelled by early trauma, leading to quickly triggered threat-based self-preservative aggression (Yakeley, 2009).

Hot aggressors often misread cues, perhaps seeing anger where others would not, feeling easily shamed. Those experiencing violence and trauma can quickly flip into sympathetic nervous system arousal, their amygdalae firing more strongly than average in response to threatening triggers (Qiao *et al.*, 2012). Reactive aggression is associated with lower attention spans, worse verbal ability, high autonomic reactivity (McLaughlin *et al.*, 2014) and low mentalising (Arsenio and Gold, 2006). We must feel relatively safe for empathy and compassion to come online; as when danger looms primitive survival responses are needed instead.

Working with 'hotter' forms of aggression can often yield more hopeful results, which was the case with Sophia. On first meeting her, I was struck by her tall angular gait, tough 'masculine' stance and threatening posture. She was the kind of young woman who rarely comes to therapy. She talked about hitting her boyfriend, was disparaging of weakness and vulnerability in anyone, including me, and fired an early warning shot by stating that she never admitted caring for anyone. She had had several major operations as an infant, the earliest when just days old, and imminent threat-based disaster was seemingly engrained in the fibres of her being.

Sophia was 17 when she arrived for psychotherapy following violent sexual enactments. Initially it was hard to decipher whether her aggression was primarily cold or reactive. She was certainly filled with core-complex anxieties and addicted to sexual and other forms of power.

Sophia had good reason to develop effective armoury against softer aspects of herself. Her early trauma was exacerbated by having three tough, macho older brothers who teased and taunted her. She had lacked parental figures who could help her manage dependency, sadness or softness and refused to show hurt, or even feel it.

Sophie had a proclivity for aggressive sexual encounters wherever, whenever and with whoever temptation arose. These derived partly from a wish for intimacy, but also a callous attack on dependency in herself or others. As is common with 'hot' aggression, she had poor impulse control, and when triggered she lost empathy, treating others as if they were there to satisfy her needs.

Not surprisingly in the transference I too was a potential 'conquest'. In an early session she flirtatiously asked if I liked her clothes, describing how by day she is mostly nearly naked, as a sports and swimming coach, describing sexual encounters and how she fancied men who were older and mysterious. I felt like potential prey. I maintained clear clarity about boundaries and my absolute refusal of her seductive manner led to us both feeling safer.

She had no respect for weak men; her boyfriend and father were ridiculed ruthlessly for their inadequacies. Her brothers all had different fathers, something they only learnt about in their teens and Sophie could not be sure who her actual father was.

As therapy proceeded, a softer side appeared. Material crept into sessions such as mentioning her sympathy for a 2-year-old cousin who she witnessed being bullied. She wondered if she was a wanted baby, whether her parents had ever loved each other, in other words whether a loving sexual encounter was possible. She talked about her shame of the scar from her early operation, something she kept hidden, and of course I thought about her hiding her emotional wounds. She could tell me how she felt different, how scared she was of darkness and of being alone.

Yet alongside softening and hope, a fear of not being in control reared its warrior-like head, banishing softness, leading to a belittling of others' vulnerability, such as her ex-boyfriend of whom she said, 'I can have him whenever I want.' If I showed sympathy for vulnerability I was dumped into the category of the soft and useless. She eulogised 'hard-as-nails' TV soap-opera characters and denigrated gentler men as 'little boys'.

Her highly armoured carapace protected her but stopped any yearned-for intimacy. If I talked about her fear of vulnerability she assumed I was joining the side of strength against weakness (hers). If I suggested that she needed me to tolerate softer aspects of her, she felt I was speaking from a position of smug superiority. Indeed, interpretations made from a too distant 'outside the ditch' place gave me, in her eyes, a steely aura, one she was all too impressed by.

One week she was late, having missed the week before, explaining nonchalantly that she had fought with her new (female) partner, then angrily, gone out and shouted at a stranger. By now she could admit when she felt let down and hurt, which was new. Some reflective functioning was developing, a buffer between the 'unthought' hurt and ensuing violent acts.

She developed a fascination for my previous patient, a girl who often left sessions crying. Sophia insisted this other patient must be 'pathetic' and 'weird'. Over time she began to ask about the tissues in the room, 'What are they were there for?' 'Who uses them?' 'Why do you put them there?' Slowly the tissues changed in her mind from weapons of torture to something else. Such tentative moves towards vulnerability were swiftly followed by a harsh re-emergence of callousness. For example, she recounted humiliating a girl she was besotted with by sleeping with the girl's best friend.

Yet something was changing, seen even in her dreamlife. This was previously full of violent nightmares but now her dreams had more narrative and softer storylines. She dreamt a blue motorbike came down a hill and hurt her new female partner and she felt contrite and worried. Earlier that week she had been tattooed with a blue devil, the same blue colour as the motorbike. This came when her partner had said that she 'loved her', and Sophie begrudgingly admitted to me that she liked this, but then acted with renewed callousness. She needed me to help her bear such soft feelings, not rubbish them. I seized such moments to talk firmly but with feeling about this. Without the firmness in my voice I was denigrated as soft and impotent; yet without the 'heartfelt' and softer tone in my voice, I had little impact. Even now, session endings were treated as if I were cruelly toying with her soft feelings. Yet our work was stirring something to life, rather like water and fertiliser can help a long-buried seed begin to grow.

After about a year she could say, 'I want to feel love, but it is best to be a bastard.' She still needed harshness to protect her fledgling softness, but less so. She bravely told me about her feelings following an abortion a few years back, and then again became aggressive to me, my job being to bear her contradictory sides.

It was another six months before a hint of tears arrived, and the backlash from this was huge, as she felt that I had humiliated her. Yet gentleness was taking root, almost despite herself. After 18 months an ending was looming, as she was preparing to go away to college. She asked what would happen with a tear in her eye, admitted not liking change, how she had kept her dentist and doctor for many years. She started to wonder about my life, 'Are you married?' 'Do you have children?'

She became flirtatious again, tempted to destroy hope rather than suffer the pain of losing closeness. She told me about an older male colleague she had seduced. I again stated, simply, that getting close here had been hard, a big risk, and maybe it would be easier to ruin this, like she has with others. I repeated what I said earlier in the therapy, that she needed to feel safe, to trust that together we could bear the excruciating feelings of being safe but close. She heard this differently now, with relief, even gratitude, showing a new capacity to bear core-complex anxieties.

She had seemed to soften by now, her body and clothes becoming more feminine, her gestures less harsh. She fought against this, saying that she hated long hair and skirts, girly things. Her voice was now less strident, maybe like a protective parent who cannot stop being overprotective even though their child has outgrown the need for this. As we neared the end of our sessions together I learnt more about her early months. She had had several serious operations in the first weeks of her life. She had been jaundiced, had an infected bowel that became gangrenous and a major part of her large intestine removed, few had thought she would live.

She now could receive empathic comments from me, which previously would have been disdainfully rebuffed. She was forming better friendships and a more trusting sexual relationship. Before the final holiday break, she could describe her wish to retaliate, by leaving therapy prematurely, just as she threatened to be unfaithful in relationships when her vulnerability was triggered. But now she was less reactive and could allow herself to stay with the upset, no longer fearful that I was smugly enjoying her weakness. I found myself feeling warmly towards her in a way that would have been unthinkable at the start.

Summary

This chapter has examined sadism, violence and aggression in children and young people, core-complex anxieties, as well as the differences between hot reactive and cold callous presentations. I have discussed the challenges of facing up to cruelty in children while holding realistic hope, keeping in mind both the victim and perpetrator in the same body. In such cases change does not come easily, but is certainly possible, and is far more likely in reactive presentations such as Sophia's, than in colder more callous ones as seen in Mick.

Chapter 11

Altruism and compassion

How they can be turned on and off

Many children and adults from tough backgrounds present with unsavoury character traits, but with help such as therapy a thawing occurs, leading to them becoming more cooperative, warm-hearted, nurturing, even altruistic and compassionate (Gilbert, 2014). Some argue that we are fundamentally a selfish not altruistic species (Dawkins, 2006). For them what looks like care is really self-motivated reciprocal altruism (Trivers, 1971), based on a 'I'll scratch your back if you'll scratch mine' philosophy. While such reciprocal altruism exists, evidence shows that genuine altruism is part of our evolutionary heritage, but requires good-enough experiences to come online. When under threat our capacity for empathy, compassion and altruism diminishes.

Those who have suffered maltreatment are often less empathic. It is no coincidence that disproportionate numbers of maltreated children act violently, are excluded from school or are in the criminal justice system. The environments they grew up in often required distrust, vigilance and anger for survival, while empathy and generosity were less useful.

Humans evolved in small hunter-gather communities where mutual trust and altruism, especially to those in one's in-group, could be life-saving. However, abusive, neglectful and traumatic environments tend to dampen altruistic traits, leading to selfishness and competitiveness instead. Altruistic capacities thrive with sufficiently safe childhoods, marked by 'good-enough' (and kind-enough) caregiving. As we see in this chapter, kind and generous traits can later develop in those initially presenting as harsh and aggressive. Selfish individualism is one aspect of human nature, but so are being kind and caring. The question is what gives rise to each.

A case: Terry

Terry, 17, came to see me for twice-weekly therapy in an NHS service. He had a troubled history. His father was unreliable, violent and often in prison. Terry was the third of four siblings, the only boy. His mother had alcohol problems, but had somehow kept the family together, mostly evading social services involvement. Terry had been a troublemaker and found studying difficult. He struggled to regulate his emotions or manage peer relationships. Despite being a favoured only boy, his upbringing was emotionally harsh, the children having to fend for themselves, with little affection to go around.

Following exclusion from school aged 9, he received 18 months of thrice-weekly therapy at the local child guidance clinic, his mother also attending fortnightly. Reports suggested that he was initially dysregulated but had settled, becoming able to play imaginatively and work through important issues. Probably this therapy helped him remain in mainstream school during adolescence.

His re-referral followed dropping out of school, drinking, getting into fights and incidences of petty crime. He was in thrall to toughness and violence and wanted to disown any vulnerability, but nonetheless was shaken by seeing where his life was heading.

Typically, early on he told me, smirking, that while playing football he had provocatively got another player sent off. He grinned on describing being threatened with a knife by the player's friend, insisting that if someone makes a fool of him he will retaliate, indeed that he had once broken a player's leg. When I suggested that he needs me to understand why he acts as he does, not agree with it, but make sense of his motives, he relaxed slightly.

Ironically, he said that such actions were his 'therapy', making him feel better. I suggested this was anti-therapy, as therapy means managing to bear difficult feelings not push them into others. He insisted that he feels better if he gets revenge, saying 'you need to get back at people, there ain't no choice, none'. I give a mock quizzical look, aware of the need to challenge him but not get into a fight. He said it is their fault. I replied, trying to gently tease, 'Oh, so if you have a bad feeling, it must be someone else's fault?' to which he retorted, slightly flummoxed, 'Well it is, isn't it?' I was realising just how much he lived in the mindset that Klein (1946) called paranoid-schizoid, with an unshakeable conviction in an 'eye for an eye' mentality.

He hated admitting weakness or incompetence, determined to project these elsewhere, including on to other racial groups and women. He often made racist comments and boasted of sexual conquests of naïve girls.

After some months though he met a girl he really liked, but his fear of dependency was excruciating. When his girlfriend was invited to a party, but not him, he deliberately invited out her best friend and was triumphant when his girlfriend was upset, saying, gloatingly, 'She has a crap time and I have a great time, and so there you are, one nil.' Yet his actions were so blatant that he had to admit feelings of neediness and jealousy to me, and was starting to understand how he projected such unwanted feelings onto others.

Over time, he became interested in softer feelings, expressing bemusement when noting the affection in his girlfriend's family. He said:

> What I do not understand is that they kiss or hug each other every day, just because she had not seen him since yesterday, well to me that's mad. I mean my dad, he would not kiss my sisters if he had been away a year.

I felt sad thinking of him growing up in such an affectionless family. He probably picked my feelings up, looked momentarily upset but quickly pushed this aside, looking angry. I noted how he often rubbished anything good and hopeful. He insisted that if this is what relationships are like, they are not for him. I said how sad I find it that he needs to belittle others to make himself feel better. I said, 'Trusting others a bit, your girlfriend or me, is hard and risky, and so it should be; not trusting was the correct life lesson to learn in your family.' He said, 'But why should I put myself on the line? It is stupid. From her I demand 100% commitment or nothing', hiding his vulnerability behind his well-oiled, tough-guy stance.

I took up how jealous he was of his girlfriend, of her family's warmth and affection. He looked sad, saying that he never had anything like that in his house. In his girlfriend's house, they had pictures of the children everywhere but in his house, there were no photos at all. I felt sadness well up in me. I said, 'Despite trying to believe in a world without caring support, you also long for it. Perhaps you hope I can help him with this?' He suddenly looked younger, somewhat shaken but touched.

In the coming months he became less angry and aggressive, but more self-critical. He told me, 'I am just a useless bastard. I have failed at everything. I will never get a job.' Seeing such self-denigrating feelings beneath the toughness suggested that he had the potential to manage more difficult feelings, although this would prove painful.

I had to walk therapeutic tightropes. I needed to show compassion, be solidly there, not buy into his self- (and other)-hatred, but also avoid sentimentality. When I pointed out his self-hating thought processes, how he rubbishes himself, how awful it must be to be on the receiving end of that, he looked perplexed, saying that he cannot understand me not being critical.

He had struggled during a therapy break, finding himself upset without realising why. He had felt self-hating and then acted nastily to his girlfriend. I asked whether he believed his vulnerability could be accepted and borne, by me, his girlfriend, eventually himself. He looked sad and said how he had spent his life determined to be strong. I said, trying to find a tone that he could tolerate, how hard it is to bear having a weaker, more vulnerable side, and entrusting that part of himself to me or anyone else. I felt momentarily deeply pessimistic, probably experiencing something of his hopelessness. I said with feeling that he really needed me to know just how desperate he feels sometimes. He again relaxed.

He was slowly taking back feelings that he habitually projected into others, but this was painful. We project for good reasons, it is much easier if it is others who are bearing difficult feelings. Slowly self-hatred and despair turned into a more self-accepting view of himself. He said, for example, 'In fact things have been all right, going great guns with me and A.' He had begun trusting his girlfriend's feelings for him. When he described how she cried because he had shown caring feelings towards her, he made a deflecting joke but in fact was moved. He particularly could not believe that her love had not diminished after he disclosed what he talks about in therapy.

As therapy progressed, with more self-reflection came more compassion, both for himself and others too. His anxiety and hyperawareness of me also diminished, and trust increased. Most strikingly, he began to do things that one could only describe as kind or caring. He started to teach younger children football. Other signs of siding with the weak and vulnerable included giving an elderly neighbour a lift to go shopping and helping a struggling young person who he worked with at weekends. He always diminished the importance of such acts, saying jokingly, for example of the old man, 'I tried to run over the old git when he was coming towards me', but such statements had lost their venom, were no longer convincing. He was genuinely becoming more caring.

This is a common pathway. As people become kinder to themselves, accepting previously disavowed and denigrated parts of themselves, they often become more altruistic. Genuine kindness for others arrives alongside kindness to the self, which of course in turn begins with kindness from others.

Human infants want to be helpful

Terry's transformation occurred after receiving experiences he lacked when young, of kindness, compassion, thoughtfulness, rather than the toughness and cynicism that was the bread and butter of his early life.

Research (Tomasello, 2009) shows that children as young as 14 months are innately helpful to adults, given the opportunity. In experimental situations when an adult feigns having a problem, such as dropping a needed object or struggling to open a cupboard, toddlers are nearly always quick to help. They read the intentions of the adults, and show a spontaneous desire to help. Such helping is intrinsically rewarding, even firing reward circuits in the brain (Moll et al., 2005).

The idea that children are naturally motivated by empathic concerns contradicts beliefs that they are primarily self-interested and need to be taught to become pro-social. In one study, babies as young as 3 months watched 3-D animations of kindly or 'nasty' figures that either 'help or hinder' another from climbing a steep hill. They demonstrably preferred the helpers to the hinderers, fully understanding each of their different 'intentions' (Hamlin et al., 2007), distinguishing helpful and unhelpful acts. Similarly, in another study 3-month-olds showed surprise when an innocent character approaches a seemingly nasty one, but not when they approach a 'good guy' (Kuhlmeier et al., 2003), clearly distinguishing pro-social and antisocial behaviours.

By 21 months toddlers generally actively reward 'helpers' and punish 'bad' puppets. Surprisingly, babies of just a few months prefer puppets that punish the bad puppets over puppets who are nice to the baddies, seemingly valuing moral acts over simple 'niceness'.

Such experiments suggest that empathy and moral sensibility naturally develop with ordinary attuned mind-minded attention. Something different occurs in chronically maltreated and neglected children who often show less empathy. By a year, children have built up considerable expectations of relationships, based on past experiences. Some children watched a scenario in which a mother and baby were climbing some steps, the baby couldn't keep up and started to cry. In one variation the mother returned for the baby, and in the other the baby was left. Securely attached children showed evident surprise when the baby was left, but the insecure children instead showed surprise when the mother returned to her children (Johnson *et al.*, 2007). Expectations of helpful behaviour are built on previous kind experiences, which in turn trigger altruistic tendencies.

However, ongoing maltreatment can inhibit these altruistic tendencies. Main and George (1985) found that most toddlers respond sympathetically to other toddlers' distress in nursery, however abused children showed little such concern and indeed could be aggressive to distressed children. More securely attached children generally show more empathy (Mikulincer *et al.*, 2005) and play well with other children, whereas conflicts increase when an insecurely attached child is involved.

Different attachment styles give rise to different responses, when the opportunity to offer help arises. Securely attached adults are likely to offer help and compassionate caregiving, those with avoidant attachments show fewer pro-social tendencies, while those with an anxious attachment, who are more self-preoccupied, are less likely to offer support from genuinely altruistic motives (Mikulincer *et al.*, 2005). It makes sense that anxious and avoidant attachment give rise to less empathy and altruism than secure attachment, given that attachment patterns are successful adaptations to early environments. In chronic abuse and maltreatment, pro-social behaviours and empathy are simply less helpful strategies.

Compassion emerges: Sophia again

I have often seen, through psychotherapy, people become softer, kinder to themselves, more caring, curious and generous to others, and live more meaningful lives. I am not sure which therapeutic factors facilitate such changes. Certainly, showing empathy is important, as is openness, curiosity and a degree of firmness. However, if I had to pick out one factor as indispensable, it would be the absence of being judgemental, or perhaps more importantly, the active presence of compassionate states of mind. Compassion does not denote a soft fluffy kindness. Rather it requires courage to stay open to our own and others' vulnerability.

When discussing sadistic states of mind in the last chapter, I introduced Sophia, who had been violent, sexually aggressive and often hurt those close to her to momentarily bolster her own moods. The only girl in the family, she had been mercilessly teased and had needed to toughen up to survive. I described how, at first, she was in thrall to violence, aggression and callousness, which protected her from painful or vulnerable feelings. With therapy she became softer, more able to give and receive love and manage the complex psychological challenges of being in a relationship, with its inevitable hurts, thwarted wishes and compromises.

My journey with Sophia required that I managed powerful projections that came flying my way. She often made me into a 'pathetic', weak or stupid person, projecting parts of herself that she could not bear. If I even had a cold I felt despised as weak and when showing ordinary care I was mocked as naïve. She brusquely rejected attempts to reach out to a soft dependent part of her. I often felt stupid and tempted to resort to a tougher more distant therapeutic stance.

I tried to remain open and compassionate. I had to work hard to be kind to the part of me that easily feels humiliated or retaliatory. Shame, a powerful social emotion, is hard to bear for any of us, but if I could not bear a bit of humiliation without resorting to aggression, then Sophia had no chance.

In time, this paid dividends. I reported in Chapter 10 how, as Sophia began to soften slightly, she said, 'I want to have loving feelings, but it is best to be a bastard and hurt others.' Like Terry, in time she began to risk being softer, kinder, even loving. This, as I have often seen, expressed itself in acts of generosity and altruism. She would babysit her older brother's children, for example, and struggled to disguise the pleasure, even love, she felt when with them. She even became compassionate towards her father, for whose weakness she previously expressed only disdain. She sat with him when he was unwell, learning about his own awful childhood, moved by stories he told.

To me, instead of being disparaging, she was almost caring on one occasion when I arrived looking unwell. After a long struggle to refuse any feelings of need, any hint of mutually caring feelings, eventually she could allow genuine warmth, albeit often disguised by teasing and an acerbic wit. She knew, and knew that I knew, that there were caring feelings between us, affectionate and even, dare I say, loving, feelings she could no longer sexualise or deny, feelings that felt like the key to her future well-being.

Fred

In Chapter 9 I described Fred, a foster child who had been shockingly abused by his stepfather. He had re-enacted violent scenes that led to him being re-traumatised and having flashbacks. I made the mistake of allowing him to re-enact traumatic events prematurely, before he had the emotional equipment to process these. I then stepped back to allow more ordinary play, for example games with balls or making structures.

Slowly he returned to imaginary play that felt different to earlier traumatic re-enactments. In one session, he wanted to go on a journey. 'Where to?' I asked. 'The Amazon', he replied. 'Ok', I said, and we made mock preparations. I was playacting a slightly older mentor. He decided we would go by bicycle, asking sweetly, 'And how far is the Amazon, six hours?'

The play felt like that of an ordinary 6-year-old, with spontaneity, engrossment and excitement. In South America we met many characters and had multiple adventures. This play lasted for several sessions. Strikingly, the characters in the stories were filled with generosity, creatures helping each other, predators being taken to task, baddies transforming into kind characters.

The play had many hopeful features. Even the idea of having an adventure and not knowing what might happen next is unusual for maltreated traumatised children who rarely risk uncertainty, let alone enjoy it. This suggested newfound faith in what life might bring, something we began to see at home too. The play was full of empathy and the ability to take others' perspectives, again new for Fred, rare in maltreated children and, as research shows, a precondition for compassionate and altruistic acts.

This allowed deeper exchanges. Fred played the role of a child kangaroo (Kanga), who in the forest met an older female kangaroo. As so often happens in foster children's play, kanga too was in foster care and the older kangaroo who was chanced upon by young Kanga was his biological mother, who was now old and hungry. He wanted the foster carer (me) to ask Kanga's biological mother whether it was ok for Kanga to stay in his new family. She said, touchingly, 'Well yes, you are doing a really nice job.' Then the foster carer checked with Kanga and they agreed to ask if the biological mother wanted to travel with them for a bit. This was very touching, demonstrating the emergence of real care, alongside an ability to mourn painful realities.

Fred's play deepened in the coming months. Games were played with toy animals, and often there was a bad, violent and uncaring parent who hurt a child. This though no longer triggered traumatic memories. In every play sequence, he introduced kind adults who would protect the child and offer a new, safe home. Fred really had internalised an idea that the world could be safe, protective and nurturing.

In one session, he re-enacted, for the first time in ages, a scene with his violent stepfather. I was nervous. Was he ready, I wondered? Could this re-traumatise him as earlier play had? This time though it was different. The stepfather was aggressive but Fred calmly used the toy phone and called the police (played by me), 'Hello, is that the police, come now, it is my stepfather, he is being violent and hurting me.' I came with other policemen and the stepfather was arrested. Then we changed roles, and I became the boy and he the policeman. As the policeman, Fred made food for the boy, and caringly put him to bed, even checking out his feelings. In my role as pretend-Fred I felt looked after by Fred when he was enacting being the policeman. I knew he now genuinely understood about being caring and being cared for. The policeman slept on the sofa and watched over the house, the atmosphere calm and safe.

In the play it was soon morning, and he told me to pretend to make a cup of tea for the policeman. Generosity and kindness were two-way in

Fred's new world. As the policeman, he said, 'Thank you. Now I have something to say to you. Have you ever heard of foster care? It is where another grown-up looks after you. They will be kind and you will feel happy there.' I played up to this, pretending to worry that I might be as badly treated as before, how could I trust a stranger? Fred as the kind policeman was clear. 'We will be watching and checking and you can always get in touch but we know that you will be looked after.' His tone was patient, reassuring and kind, all qualities he now knew deeply inside himself –very different from the Fred I had met a few years back.

Pathological kindness?

Some forms of caring of others derives from less positive motives. You might remember Grace from Chapter 4. Her attachment style was primarily ambivalent, she had had a chaotic background in which, in order to feel safe, she needed to look after those around her.

The cost of this was that she was often far too nice, not believing that her real self, with ordinary feelings like upset, worry or anxiety, could be tolerated by others. A major job of therapy was to help her believe that she did not have to constantly look after others. People like Grace are often genuinely likeable, popular and good to have around. She was expert in making others feel good, including me.

While for other children mentioned in this chapter, the move towards being helpful and kind was central to the road to recovery, this is not the case for children like Grace. For them, being helpful to others can mean being unhelpful to themselves, enacting compliant niceness rooted in keeping safe, a very different state of mind from the self-compassion or other-compassion that I had begun to see in Terri, Sophia and Fred.

Conclusions

Empathy, compassion and altruism tend to emerge given 'good-enough' (Winnicott, 1953) early caregiving. Altruistic tendencies have roots in early life, even seen in babies. On receiving sensitive attuned mind-minded attention, infants learn to trust, be interested in people's thoughts and feelings, read intentions and want to participate in cooperative group-life. Such traits often get turned off in trauma and maltreatment.

From about 9 months old, capacities to understand other minds grow apace. By 14 months, most can pass the classic 'mirror-recognition' test. Here, one places a blob of 'rouge' on an infant's face and children 'pass' this test if they recognise, looking in a mirror, that the face with the rouge is theirs. Interestingly, Dutch research showed that toddlers who responded empathically to another's sadness were the children who had already passed the 'rouge' mirror self-recognition test (Bischof-Köhler, 2012), whereas those who failed the test were less sympathetic. Capacities for understanding one's own and other minds, for empathy and the desire to help others, tend to develop together. However they develop much less in traumatised children and adults.

As we have seen, capacities to defer gratification and self-regulate are seen more in securely attached children and less in traumatised ones. In fact the ability to delay gratification predicts many outcomes right into adulthood, such as the likelihood of holding down a job, managing a stable romantic relationship or negotiating good friendships, to name but a few (Mischel, 2014). Deferred gratification and altruism tend to come together.

The model of social and emotional development used in this book assumes an inbuilt human propensity for relationships from birth onwards, what Trevarthen (2001) called having a 'companion in meaning-making'. This is in line with Bråten (1998), who considered infants to be born 'alterocentric' rather than Piaget's (1965) 'egocentric' infant. This suggests that selfishness is neither more nor less natural than altruism, but that it increases with stress and threat.

Of course, all 'ordinary' children, indeed any of us, are capable of sadism and nastiness. Nonetheless being helpful, interested in other people, following social rules and wanting to be part of a moral order develops more 'naturally' than is sometimes thought.

However, maltreatment, anxiety and stress, as well as an increasingly stressful, competitive and individualistic culture, undermines this. Therapeutic work, as I hope the accounts here show, can counter such experiences and facilitate compassionate states of mind, actions and even compassionate cultures.

As Gordon (1999) emphasised, psychotherapy is an 'ethical' endeavour, ineluctably linked to what we hope for in human relationships. When it goes well, therapeutic work leads to more empathic, thoughtful, self-reflective and playful people with increased capacities for self-regulation, better able to relate to others, with more compassion and humanity. This is what we saw in Terry, Sophia and Fred, who all softened, became less self-critical, and more accepting of vulnerability in themselves and others. This gave rise to the growth of generous, kind and altruistic behaviour to others and a richer, more fulfilled life, with more ease and well-being and more interpersonal rewards. That should give us hope for a better world.

Chapter 12

Addiction, tech and the web
New dangers hijacking old systems

Digital worlds, new challenges

These days the Internet and digital technology confront us with challenges unknown to previous generations of professionals and parents. Few doubt that technologies are changing lives, even if the jury remains out on its proven impacts. Cyber-related issues are growing apace, nearly all children and young people being affected, especially the most vulnerable who face new risks.

Typical was 14-year-old Mitchell. He was living with his father, his mother having tragically died of cancer three years earlier after a long illness. His father had then retreated, working long hours, unable to process the death. Mitchell's school work deteriorated and he became increasingly withdrawn. He moved in with his paternal grandmother, his father visiting regularly. Mitchell withdrew into his bedroom, immersed in computer games, and little could entice him away. He was increasingly unconfident anyway and socialising had little allure. When he transitioned to secondary school he struggled to cope with the hurly burly of a huge school and barely feeling held in mind by any of the adults.

It makes sense to think of Mitchell's gaming as addictive. Such games offer multiple rewards, hooking players with never-ending prospects of ascending levels and higher scores. We have known about the brain states involved for over 60 years. When rats found that pulling a lever stimulated the nucleus accumbens, a brain area central for dopamine release, they prioritised such pleasure-seeking over everything, including sex and food (Olds and Milner, 1954). Something similar can happen with games and other forms of technology over-use.

In my youth, bored kids, including myself, spent hours in repetitive solitary games. I, for example, played imaginary football tournaments with dice for hours. Even when friends came around I could struggle for a while to leave my game, although as soon as I did I had no regrets.

Such games were used in part to fend off difficult feelings like loneliness, anxiety, poor confidence or other emotional difficulties. Compared to old fashioned more innocent games, today's gaming environment has built-in tricks that hook users in extraordinarily sophisticated ways.

Video games deliver a steady stream of rewards to keep us online, with the lure of almost infinite levels to climb. They work on the powerful principle of variable rewards, which is also how social media keeps people hooked. If we know that putting X into a slot machine always results in receiving a Y, then we will do this when wanting a Y, but not constantly. If putting that same amount in might result in a huge range of potential rewards, but we never know quite what, then it keeps us coming back to check. This is what happens with Instagram, Twitter, Facebook and other media. When life is difficult, as Mitchell's was, such potential rewards can trump real relationships and social connections, which ideally would be life's main reward.

In Mitchell's case, it was not targeting his addiction that made the difference, but rather taking seriously the emotional gulf in his life. In family sessions, with Mitchell's father alongside his grandmother, space was made for Mitchell's feelings. Early tentative sessions explored his mother's illness, death and the feelings they had all struggled to face. It was imperative to help his father to bear his own sense of loss. He spent early sessions tense, sitting near the door, clutching his phone, ready to retreat, warding off overwhelming grief and sadness. In one session, Mitchell reminded dad of Mitchell's mum, saying, 'It is like, well I look at Mitch and I just see, just see ... [his eyes started to tear up and his voice choked], oh god, I just see Jan [Mitchell's mum].' The whole room was in tears, including me. Afterwards the feeling of relief was palpable, there was a new stillness and sense of closeness.

Dad began spending more time with Mitchell, who in turn seemed happier. Mitchell had felt rejected by his father but was now experiencing being thought about, liked and indeed loved. He spent less time on his computer. Dad made plans to move in and to get a place together. Dad also had met a new partner who Mitchell seemed to get on with. Positive change was unusually quick in this case. Mitchell began to feel more confident, started to socialise and, as we often see, his schoolwork improved.

Mitchell had had a reasonably good start, with several good years with a loving mother before losing her, retaining a deep sense of his lovability and that life could be ok. This is often not true of more vulnerable children who succumb addictively to the lure of digital technology. Mitchell had been using gaming to ward off difficult feelings, but we caught Mitchell's situation in time, before the technology had got its claws completely into him.

Sexting

Katie, 13, had recently stopped seeing her first boyfriend, Dom. They were in the same class and she had previously counted him as a friend. Her parents did not approve of her having a boyfriend, especially one from a 'rougher' neighbourhood. Katie though did not feel ready for the kind of sexual enactments she felt pressured into. Dom, like many of his age, pushed through low confidence by adopting a masculinity gleaned crudely from pornography. While Dom's machismo was defending against his vulnerability, it pushed Katie into a corner. She was besotted with Dom, 'madly in love' she said, but felt out of her comfort zone and ended the relationship.

Dom was hurt and took revenge by sending out revealing pictures of Katie. Within minutes these were widely distributed. When she realised what had happened, Katie was distraught and could barely breathe, feeling deeply shamed, not wanting to leave the house.

Such cybertrauma (Knibbs, 2016) or cyberbullying (Zych et al., 2017), is increasingly common and often linked with worrying outcomes, even suicidality in serious cases (Kowalski et al., 2014).

Luckily, Katie was also from a loving, supportive family and had good resources to draw from, in herself, family and friends In fact, it was Dom who suffered. He was punished, shamed, the episode being taken seriously at senior levels of the school where strict guidelines were put in place. Dom was excluded from school, and new lessons were rolled out, airing issues of sexting, pornography and digital technology.

Katie's case is unusual, especially in terms of the enlightened attitude of her school. Often it is the more vulnerable children who suffer most. One profoundly neglected vulnerable young man, Majid, had a history of being bullied in school, often in sadistic sexualised ways. For example, he was forced into a form of sexual contact with an animal, which was photographed, the pictures going viral. He also became mixed up with a gang who used him as a drug mule. When he tried to withdraw, they threatened him violently and the situation was so dangerous that the police suggested Majid not only change schools but even move cities. These days, images and reputations follow people across the globe and into perpetuity.

Possessing pictures, such as of Katie or Majid, is in effect carrying child pornography, which carries legal sanctions. Perhaps more importantly, lives can get ruined by such acts, and as in Majid's case, it is those who are struggling anyway, who have had little social support or care at home, who suffer the most.

Marsha and social media

New media offer so much that is exciting, including instant social networking and social support. Yet there are downsides, and again the most at risk are the already vulnerable.

Typical was Marsha, 13, who became inadvertently involved in a sexting scenario that threatened her reputation. An only child adopted from Russia at the age of 7 by a single mother, when young she was both seriously neglected and exposed to sexualised behaviour. She struggled in friendships, felt lonely, emotionally flat and deadened. She managed cravings for an intimacy she also feared by engaging in inappropriate online encounters with men, which she found exciting.

In Marsha I saw some common features often also seen in males addicted to pornography. She presented in an emotionally withdrawn, lifeless way. Her potential life force, what Freud would have called her 'libido', sexual or otherwise, seemed only to come alive via the excitement of online encounters. Otherwise she could not express or even know that she had desires.

Marsha indulged in worrying Internet activity in a way that meant she would inevitably get caught, provoking her mother who then became despairing and angry with her. This pattern became a form of sadomaso-chistic enactment in itself, allowing her to avoid real intimacy with her mother while keeping her close and 'on her case', in classic core-complex style (Glasser, 1992).

After being caught posting naked pictures of herself online, her technology was removed. Ostensibly, consciously, she wanted this and was pleased to be protected. However, forces bigger than her conscious will took over, especially at stressful periods, such as exam times or when a friendship went wrong. Then she would do almost anything to acquire technology, fuelling what seemed like an addiction. She would scour the house ghostlike in the night, find old laptops and smartphones, communicating online with unknown people. She even stole friend's phones to do this.

Many men communicating with girls like Marsha are using false names, grooming several children simultaneously, yet making each child feel special and unique. The underlying issues are not new, in Marsha's case the paucity of love, attention and kindness in her early life and the exposure to exciting sexuality, giving rise to a personality ripe for such exploitation. However, for Marsha, as for many addicted tech users, the technology allows them to be exploited with an ease impossible in the past.

Marsha had to slowly learn to bear the feelings stirred up in intimate human encounters, including in her therapy. As more genuine emotional relating became possible, her core-complex anxieties could slowly be relinquished. She could be more vulnerable, especially with her mother and therapist. She began to crave attention, and believe in its possibility, but this also felt like a huge risk. She would quickly retreat when she felt spurned, or be manipulative and controlling to get the attention she craved. Therapy can be a kind of practice for life, a place to learn about emotions and one's inner life, where intimacy and trust in genuine closeness can be experimented with, and evolve.

The process of becoming emotionally healthier for young people like Marsha is slow, with many false positives. Powerful feelings of loss and need can get stirred up, such as in gaps between sessions. As Marsha learnt to bear such feelings, and as hopeful aspects of her personality developed, her symptoms began to abate. As Marsha began to believe in her likeability and her ability to be known emotionally, she relied less on old patterns, her desires no longer enacted in such worrying ways.

With many pornography users, we see something similar. Addictive symptoms worsen with increased vulnerability, and in crises. What they, like Marsha, lack is a good internal object to rely on, one to help them bear and come through difficulty, to help them trust that things can work out well enough in the end. Of course, there needs to be weaning from the technology too. While someone is coming off a drug like cocaine one does not leave piles of the white powder around their home. The same applies to the temptations of technology. However, this is not enough. Most worrying use of technology is a turning away, from challenging feeling states, from human relationships and intimacy. When the powerful emotions linked to intimacy can be borne, addictive tendencies diminish.

Pornography: a different kind of story

Later I discuss a more conventional case of pornography addiction, but now I introduce Dillon, whose relationship with pornography was unusual. By 16 he had a child pornography conviction. On the surface, little about his past would have suggested this. His history was relatively straightforward, without obvious abuse or trauma, apart from mild bullying by an older half-brother, and a somewhat fraught parental divorce when he was 9 years old.

What was different about Dillon was the nature of his sexual desires. He had never found girls or boys of his own age attractive, going cold at the thought of sexual encounters with them. He was often aroused in public situations, such as swimming baths, or even buses and trains. He was good-looking, girls his age often approach him and he had unsuccessfully tried to become involved with them, desperately wanting to be 'normal'. He had only ever felt arousal for prepubescent girls, but desperately wished he was not this way.

Dillon found himself managing these feelings by looking at images online, often relatively innocuous ones, such as in clothing catalogues. Then he discovered the Dark Web, where worrying and illegal sites could be accessed. Here he found pornography depicting sexual encounters with girls of the age he was aroused by, sometimes involving overt sexual acts with adult men. This discovery filled Dillon with relief and pleasure. Which might sound shocking but these images expressed his desires, and left him feeling less alone. Such pornography use lessened his fantasising about real live prepubertal girls.

Dillon's paedophilia seemed like a primary sexual orientation, rather like some people primarily relate as heterosexual, gay or lesbian. This is rare, but well described in the therapeutic literature (Wood, 2013). Many paedophilic men are also interested in people of other ages or genders, but not Dillon. He was not sexually active, doing everything in his power to avoid contact with children he felt aroused by. Having used child pornography to help manage his desires, he was ensnared into sharing images and was prosecuted for possessing and distributing illegal images.

Many men who undertake paedophilic acts, or have sexual fantasies about children, were abused as children or inappropriately exposed to high levels of sexual stimulation. Unlike Dillon, their paedophilia is 'secondary', not a primary sexual orientation. Sexual enactments towards children by such abused men can be a way of giving others a taste of their own experience of being abused. Often, if such initial traumas are worked through in therapy, and links made to when and why their feelings and impulses are triggered, the re-enactments lessen. Many adults who were abused as children do relate sexually to people of their own age, in a way that Dillon never could.

Dillon's case is tragic. We do not know why or how he ended up as he did, whether this was a biological inheritance, a brain wiring issue or something yet to be discovered. For him, child pornography, with the unsavoury exploitative features that he understood, offered him an opportunity to experience what he believed was his genuine sexuality in a way he never could in real life.

Dillon worked hard in therapy. He was low in confidence, full of shame, spending hours in his bedroom alone to avoid being besieged by desires for girls on the street. Family holidays in the sun were his biggest nightmare. Much of his therapy was geared to developing self-compassion and learning to accept himself. He expended huge amounts of energy trying to push away his desires, hating himself for having them. Like the classic advice that is bound to fail of 'don't think about polar bears', the denied and disavowed inevitably pops back up.

With Dillon, I tried to stay with his feelings and fantasies, getting to really know them in all their granularity. Interspersing psychodynamic work and mindfulness, he learnt to explore his feelings and fantasies in a titrated way, to move between explorations of his sexual thoughts and focusing on his immediate body sensations, and his breath. We stayed a lot with the body sensations he experienced, both when anxious and when aroused. Over time this yielded remarkable results. He became able to bear and stay with his thoughts and feelings, even of sexual desire for girls while in public, without them taking him over and without feeling at risk of acting on them. Finding that he could actively ground himself by focusing on his body states was liberating and transformational.

I was surprised at how he took heart and practised mindfulness regularly. Dillon also had a slightly paranoid bent. He was convinced, for example, that the police were going to return to arrest him at any time. He was also certain that he had failed his exams, and nothing could dissuade him of this. In time though he could watch such thoughts and feelings come and go and not be triggered by them, just as classic mindfulness suggests. He could find a place outside the previously overwhelming thoughts and sexual fantasies. When triggered into a panicky state or fantasy he could step back, watch the thoughts arise and disappear, become aware of his body sensations in response to these, such as fast heart rate or shallow breathing, and then find a way back to calmer breath. This was never about avoiding his feelings, but rather embracing and bearing them, something that mindfulness and psychoanalysis share. Dillon eventually left therapy to go to university, confident that he could manage in the outside world, no longer plagued by self-hatred and shame.

Science and research

We have seen how poor early experiences lead to problems with emotional regulation and interpersonal relationships. High levels of technology use can exacerbate such symptoms, leading to shorter concentration spans, less ability to ignore temptation, more impulsivity, all also linked with poorer relationships. The real external world of instant gratification, fast food, one-click purchases, immediate downloads and instantaneous communications exacerbates this.

While the research remains hotly contested, some evidence suggests that, for example, high video game usage, social media use and even TV watching, are linked to shorter attention spans and quicker arousal levels. Chicken and egg are hard to unpick, as self-regulation and emotional ease come with good relationships and attuned parenting (Fumero *et al.*, 2018) and presumably children left in front of screens get less good parenting. Attachment style seems to be a mediator here, those who are more secure are less in danger (Roberts and David, 2016) and, not surprisingly, if people are more anxious, or have less sense of control over their lives, they turn to technology more (Lee *et al.*, 2018).

As Turkle (2012), Carr (2011) and others have found, over-using digital technology leads to poorer concentration and increased distractedness. So-called multi-tasking lowers performance and working memory and, of course, multi-tasking is a myth; we might switch from task to task more speedily, but do each less well, our brains being incapable of doing several things at once.

Internet use, like any tool-use, changes our brains. However, the paradox is that such brain plasticity leads to habitual behaviour patterns that are hard to shift. Carr (2011) argues that speedy, skimming mentalities are taken into social interactions, undermining empathy in relationships.

Bigger controversies centre around the ever-increasing use of video games. Some have argued that such games increase impulsivity and lower concentration (Gentile *et al.*, 2012), while other studies suggest little effect (Pan *et al.*, 2018). It is again unclear if this is causation or simply correlation, as impulsive children often play more video games, and children who play more video games become more impulsive.

Perhaps most importantly, the risks of all these technologies are greater for some than others. Emotional instability, introversion and impulsiveness increase the risk of dependency on technologies (Roberts *et al.*, 2015). As we have seen throughout this book, good relationships, secure attachment and self-compassion all come from better relationships, giving rise to valuing people rather than 'things', intrinsic rather than extrinsic rewards (Kasser, 2003).

There are dangers of embracing a Luddite fear of the new. Many games are designed to increase valued skills such as concentration (Oei and Patterson, 2013) and logical thinking, (Graf *et al.*, 2009). Serious neuroscientists have been designing technologies that enhance mindfulness (Sliwinski *et al.*, 2017), and other positive traits such as emotional regulation (Griffiths *et al.*, 2017).

Eagleman (2011) has suggested that what he calls *pre-frontal workouts* can train the 'muscles' of the regulatory and reflective areas of the brain. Various forms of neurofeedback and computer-assisted psychotherapies, such as with avatars (Leff *et al.*, 2014), are showing hopeful results. Using technologies such as EEG scanners and heart-rate monitors, subjects can now get 'real-time' feedback, enabling them to shift brain and autonomic nervous system patterns.

Yet, alongside such technologies' potential for enhancing emotional well-being, we are seeing an increase in technology-fuelled presentations and vulnerable children and young people with poorer relationships and less secure attachments are the most likely to succumb to technology's worst effects, such as Internet pornography.

A case of excessive pornography use: Mano

Mano, a late adolescent who moved to the UK with refugee parents at 8 years old, was struggling in school and spending hours watching pornography alone in his room, masturbating up to 18 times a day. The pornography that he watched was becoming increasingly violent, although still legal.

His background was not straightforward. His parents were both regular churchgoers in an evangelical congregation. His mother came from a tough family, suffering much verbal abuse in childhood. His father had been quite absent in Mano's early years and when present used excessive physical chastisement. Both parents came from backgrounds of migration and ethnic discrimination over generations. As a young boy Mano had ADHD-like symptoms, being fidgety, jumpy, unable to concentrate. He told of teachers tying one of his legs to a chair so he would stay sitting down.

He was a vigilant young man. When hearing any noise outside, his mind left the therapy to attend to expected danger. He often had fantasies about the therapy room being broken into, once saying, as he looked up at a window that had rattled, 'I know exactly what I would do if someone tried to climb through, I have planned how I would defend myself', explaining the martial arts moves he would enact.

Mano had not witnessed much violence himself, despite his parents having to leave their country of origin hurriedly. His paranoid thinking came via his parents' states of mind, possibly from secondary trauma. His father had been subjected to violence and ethnic persecution. In addition, on arrival in the UK Mano had been bullied in school.

He was vigilant to the tiniest changes in the room, such as a book being moved or something new on my desk. He found relaxation almost impossible, needing to be constantly active, although paradoxically at the cost of not doing anything well. Hence, despite a bright mind, he was failingly academically.

While such compulsive pornography use and masturbation is increasingly common in young men, some, like Mano, have more of a proclivity for addictive behaviours. He often gorged on unhealthy food, over-indulged in gaming and also occasionally stole on an impulsive whim.

Mano was quite popular in school, although somewhat isolated, as the religious school his parents had chosen was far from where they lived, limiting ordinary social interactions that might have helped resist screen-based temptations.

Mano's issues can be understood from many angles, perhaps most obviously his lifelong struggle with emotional and bodily regulation. He was likeable but not restful to be with. His leg would shake often as he spoke, his attention darting around, his mind as jumpy as his legs. I often wanted to do what a male therapist simply cannot do, put a hand on one of his to calm him down. I did sometimes suggest he take a deep breath alongside me. I felt what he needed, and had lacked, was a calming, caring parental presence.

His mother reported high levels of anxiety while pregnant and in his early months. Probably Mano was born predisposed for stress, given how maternal stress affects the developing foetus (Music, 2016). His mother suffered post-natal depression, reporting that he was hard to soothe. She was not especially psychologically minded, almost definitely unable to help him make sense of his experience in a soothing, calming way.

In such environments infants experience physiological signs of distress but cut off from bodily signals of this, which otherwise feel overwhelming. Many children and adults with similar presentations act a lot with their bodies, such as in sexual acting out or violence, but paradoxically are also extremely unaware of their body states. Mano too had poor interoceptive capacities, with little ability to recognise emotions or body states.

I adopted a more psychoeducational approach than usual. I thought that Mano would benefit from making basic links between his behaviours, impulses and their triggers. Initially his emotional vocabulary and range of known feeling states was minimal, mainly consisting of describing himself as cool or good (his positive affect states) or 'pissed' or shit (his negative emotional range). There were few nuances to build on.

'What has been happening?' I asked in one session several months in. Mano looked uneasy and then with something of a smirk told me that yesterday he 'wanked' nearly all afternoon. 'It's been bad', he said, but I felt that he was pleased, triumphant, the 'fuck-it button' victorious (Nathanson, 2016). Often, I asked how he felt and he told me what he had been doing rather than describe a feeling. Trying to make sense of what had emotionally driven him to masturbatory acting out was difficult.

In one session, at a noise of someone coming down the nearby stairs he jolted, looking around as if preparing for danger. I asked what was happening in his body in that moment, could he feel his heart beat, was it different to usual? He said, as often, 'I don't know'. I asked him to put his hand on his chest and feel his heart, which he did, almost to placate me, but became a little interested. It was of course beating quite fast. I suggested he keep his hand there and see if he could feel what happens in the next few minutes. He did and was surprised to note that he felt his heart rate slow with his breath.

As Damasio (2012) helped us understand, emotions are body states that can be 'read', if we have the mental equipment with which to read them. With Mano, I diverted from my normal psychodynamic stance, spending time guiding him through some mindfulness-based body-awareness exercises. It was fascinating how, when there were noises elsewhere in the clinic, he noted a tensing of his body or his pulse quickening. This was the beginning of making links between external triggers like a door closing loudly and a body state, which might be called a feeling state, such as anxiety. I asked, 'It might sound daft to you but when you reacted then, could we say you were anxious, or at least unsettled?' Mano almost looked interested, albeit still loath to ascribe emotional labels to himself.

I became braver in my adventures into guided techniques. I had felt stumped by his insistence that he had no clue as to why he was masturbating so much, insisting he just 'liked it'. Those few moments of pleasure when he ejaculated, he claimed, made life worthwhile. He craved this sensation like a junkie craved their next hit.

This makes sense in terms of what we know about addictive processes. In all addictions, whether drugs, gambling, shopping, alcohol or pornography, the dopaminergic system is triggered. Key areas of such brain circuitry, such as the ventral striatum, are more activated at even the sight of a cue of their addiction, such as a laptop for a porn user (Brand *et al.*, 2016), or the bottle for the alcoholic (Kraus *et al.*, 2016).

Worryingly, in pornography we see habituation, people getting used to images that then become less stimulating, driving them to watch more exciting content, often violent or illegal. High pornography use in young men can also lead to sexual problems such as erectile dysfunction (Park *et al.*, 2016). In addition porn use seems implicated in lowering the capacity to delay gratification (Negash *et al.*, 2016), and lessening activation of brain circuitry involved with empathy and executive functions.

Our dopaminergic system evolved for good reasons. It drives us towards what we need to survive and reproduce, such as sex and food. Yet this system can be hijacked by modern technology in a way that evolution has not prepared us for. Most of what modern humans feel is as ancient as our species, including negative emotions such as sadness, anxiety or grief. Alluringly, technology offers the false hope of taking such feelings away, promising respite from pain or difficulty with new exciting allurements.

Mano had been gloriously unaware of what triggered his addictions. It took a long period of guided practices, such as becoming aware of his breath and body sensations, before he could become stiller, learn to link his bodily states and emotions and then link such emotions to his drives towards pornography or over-eating. Thankfully Mano was keen to learn about himself and curb habits that he knew were unhealthy.

We know clinically, and from research (Grubbs *et al.*, 2015), that often people turn towards pornography when in distress. In people like Mano, distress can bypass the conscious experiencing mind, short cutting the possibility of bearing and processing the triggering feelings. Instead in a flash we see enactments, such as turning towards an addictive habit. For Mano, change meant slowing down reactivity to witness and then stay with the initial experience that he was fleeing. For example, I would ask what happened just before he turned on pornography. He eventually started to notice triggers, often as simple as just losing at a computer game. Then in time he could start to stay with the feelings stirred up by such triggers.

Luckily, Mano enrolled on an eight-week mindfulness training course. He became increasingly interested in his body states and even began to do yoga and other body-based practices. This though would have been insufficient without an experience of another, me, staying with his experiences, showing interest and empathy for his states of mind and emotion and not shirking how his mind could trick him. Mano in time started to relinquish the pornography as he entered an intimate and fulfilling sexual relationship. In this period, he developed other capacities. For example, he started to read novels voraciously, itself a helpful thing, enhancing concentration, self-regulation and empathy (Kidd *et al.*, 2016). He started to gravitate towards young people who were more emotionally literate, forming real friendships. In effect, he was developing the kind of capacities we see in secure attachment relationships. At the time of leaving therapy, he was in a stable relationship, had lost at least 30 pounds in weight and had not masturbated for several months.

Emotional regulation and impulsivity

Many common clinical presentations feature difficulties in emotional regulation. Mano was typical, and had little sense of his emotions. Of course no one can regulate emotions they are not aware of having. I see this often in traumatised hypervigilant children who have less access to prefrontal brain areas central for empathy, emotional regulation and self-reflection. In traditional Freudian language, such patients might be thought of as controlled by *id* impulses but having little ego functioning (Solms and Panksepp, 2012).

Much research shows the link between being able to defer gratification and better later-life outcomes. Robert Mischels (2014), who invented the famous marshmallow experiment, found in follow-ups some 40 years later that those who could delay gratification as toddlers were more likely in adulthood to be in good relationships, holding down a job and good friendships. Similarly a study (Slutske *et al.*, 2012) of over 1,000

3-year-olds found that when they reached adulthood the most restless, inattentive, oppositional and moody children were over twice as likely to be addicted to gambling. Interestingly neither IQ nor socio-economic status were anywhere near as predictive.

Self-control in children predicts scores in maths, reading, vocabulary and SATS tests (Sektnan *et al.*, 2010), and is far more predictive of exam results than IQ (Duckworth *et al.*, 2011). Another study of over 1,000 children followed until the age of 32 (Moffitt *et al.*, 2011) found that early self-control predicted physical health, substance dependence, financial success and criminal offending, again irrespective of IQ and social class. These are powerful results.

The dangers posed by digital technology are much higher for vulnerable children. Luckier children have emotionally sensitive attachment figures who can empathise with them, helping to manage difficult experiences such as frustration or anxiety, promoting self-regulation, empathy and emotional regulation (Kochanska and Kim, 2012). Secure attachment is predictive of effortful control (Meins and Russell, 2011), even if temperament also plays a role. Those who have rarely been empathised with tend to struggle to regulate emotions and are more vulnerable to the lure of technology.

Most impulsive behaviour starts for defensive reasons, often as attempts to manage stress, trauma or uncertainty. However, such behaviours can become addictive and there are plentiful forms of addictions to choose from these days. I hope to have shown in my clinical descriptions that for the more vulnerable, such as Mano, Mitchell and Marsha, technology can cause serious problems, but the root of these issues lies deeper, in their histories, emotional lives, attachment relationships and poor sense of well-being. Sometimes we must address the addiction head-on, but often addictions lose their power as people become happier, less anxious, more confident, cared for and, indeed, caring.

Chapter 13

Freeing the scapegoat by containing not blaming

Thoughts on schools-based therapeutic work (with Becky Hall)

Introduction: who is our client?

This chapter explores how to work at the most effective level of professional systems, something I had to ponder deeply while setting up therapeutic services in over 30 schools. There can be an unhelpful fit between the idea that a child has a problem, and the search for a solution that focuses on the child. This danger is exacerbated because most therapeutic training focuses on individual work, while schools often struggle to remember that a child's issues may begin elsewhere, perhaps in the family network or even the school system.

If a child misbehaves, is unhappy or aggressive, then people often assume that the problem is 'in the child' and our job is to 'cure them'. However, with complex cases, work is needed at several levels of the system, with parents, teachers and professional networks. This can be a challenge when staff are under huge pressure and hope therapists will 'take away and sort out' problem children.

Difficult-to-manage children mean much tougher work for teachers, and it is easier to see a child as naughty, disturbed, possibly needing medication, than to think about the grim realities of children's histories and life circumstances. However, understanding a child's life situation often softens teachers' views of even the most challenging children.

Some examples

One pupil, Marshall, was interrupting classes, provoking other children and spitting at his teacher. He was referred to the psychotherapist who, on meeting the family, uncovered a precarious home situation with a seriously ill mother and an unreliable father. We worked with the family and involved social services. However, probably most useful was relaying our understanding of Marshall's predicament to his overwhelmed teacher. She became moved by Marshall's plight, understanding in a new way the vulnerability beneath Marshall's aggressive defences. This teacher's newly sympathetic, softer attitude led, in turn, to an improvement in Marshall's behaviour and learning.

It often pays to meet the parents, even of adolescents, rather than offer individual work too quickly. Shirley, 13, previously a model pupil, had recently stopped doing homework. When questioned by her concerned form tutor, she was initially non-committal and then insolent. A referral to the therapist was made, but Shirley was as disparaging to the therapist as to her teacher. The parents were contacted and offered a meeting. We learnt from her tearful mother that her own mother (Shirley's grandmother), who Shirley was close to, had suffered a stroke and suddenly needed constant care. Shirley's mother was away a lot, and distracted, able to offer little to Shirley and her younger brother.

The father too was affected by his wife's absences, bravely admitting how abandoned he felt by his wife, feeling awkward becoming the primary caretaker for his adolescent daughter. Furthermore, both parents had misunderstood Shirley's increasing independence. She was seeing more friends, being less affectionate, leaving both parents feeling less needed. Couple sessions were offered. We discussed the challenges of parenting adolescents, how to allow independence but remain 'present to be left' by teenagers who still need more parental attention than they admit.

Arrangements were made for Shirley's mother to be home more, and the couple became closer again, prioritising regular family times. Shirley initially baulked at this, but was in fact relieved. She joined some later meetings, but by then was settled again, her year tutor no longer concerned. Interestingly, her brother had been referred to the local child and adolescent mental health services (CAMHS) after starting to cause trouble in primary school, yet by the time the clinic contacted the family, the situation had calmed. The work with the parents in Shirley's school seemingly had a 'knock-on' effect on her brother's behaviour.

Sometimes the therapist's role is to contain anxiety, as in Shirley's case, but it can also be to increase anxiety in a system, especially in cases of risk. One teaching assistant was anxious about a student's bleak pictures, full of relentlessly dark images of death and destruction. This had gone unnoticed by an art teacher who was more concerned with drawing technique. After consulting with the child psychotherapist, further exploration uncovered a severely depressed adolescent who had self-harmed and needed a psychiatric referral. Such interventions not only help the pupil but also generate understanding of mental health issues that can be applied to other children.

Therapeutic work in schools often involves deconstructing discourses about what constitutes a 'problem'. Children can be labelled as 'bad', 'unmanageable', 'unstable', even 'dangerous'. Yet when we can bear, contain and make sense of complex feelings such as fear, anger or hurt, in both pupils and staff, a child can be seen as sad rather than bad, hurt as well as angry, distressed rather than malevolent, needing support not exclusion. We aim to facilitate environments where children feel genuinely held in mind, 'at home' in themselves and the institution.

Mistakenly, I think, we send our least experienced therapists into schools. This is complex work requiring experience and professional authority, including communicating across agencies and sharing information with teachers and a range of professionals.

Effective therapeutic workers need excellent communication skills to help staff make sense of the children in their care. An understanding of child development, neuroscience and attachment also helps. Therapists need to spot psychiatric or child protection risk and recognise typical presenting issues such as ADHD, autism, depression, PTSD or phobias, and know the best ways of working with these. This is skilled work.

Particularly important is helping staff make sense of, and bear, the powerful emotions stirred up in them. The feelings that psychotherapists take in their stride as the meaningful bread and butter of our work, such as dependency, rivalry, envy, anger or despair, can be hard feelings for teachers to accept in pupils, and in themselves. However, it is surprisingly transformative when school staff can tolerate and find meaning in such primitive emotional states.

A simple example was a teacher who became dispirited and angry when a favourite pupil became sullen and withdrawn. This excellent teacher, feeling hurt, withdrew, not realising how the pupil struggled when he had given attention to a new pupil. This realisation alone was enough to improve the atmosphere between them.

A particularly successful model is Jackson's (2008) use of work discussion groups, whether for senior staff, head teachers or support staff. These enable staff to understand children differently, to process feelings that otherwise can get enacted, helping institutional dynamics shift and even reducing staff sickness and turnover.

In a climate of ever-increasing demands and targets, there is less room for thoughtfulness and more temptation to act precipitately. Hence the importance of helping staff process their powerful reactions to pupils, so that what might be perceived as 'misbehaviour', arousing anger and frustration, might be understood more sympathetically in terms of a child's history or current life situation. Such work can take place informally, by the staffroom kettle or in corridors, as well as more formally in groups.

Courtney: the escape of a scapegoat

In one school a new service was greeted with several referrals of children with challenging behaviour. The first boy referred was offered treatment but was permanently excluded before we had even contacted the parents. The next child on the list was soon also excluded. We spotted a pattern, whereby a child was seen as being not only 'disruptive' and a 'problem', but as 'the' problem in the school. A belief arose about a toxic presence (the bad child) contaminating an otherwise healthy system. As often, the projections hung neatly on hooks that fitted all too well pupils from complex backgrounds who genuinely had serious emotional issues but were nonetheless scapegoated.

The next *unmanageable* child was 7-year-old Courtney. She had tantrums, often cried for her mother, was volatile, hit out at other children, struggled to cope with transitions and was underachieving academically. She often wore sexualised clothes, such as tight jeans and short tops. Social services were involved, and her father had been in prison.

We met with Courtney's parents, a white working-class couple in their mid-thirties who lived on a run-down estate. There had been many family crises, including multiple tragic bereavements. In our preliminary meeting, the mother talked without pause, while the father anxiously paced the room, and it was difficult to end punctually. We learnt of an extremely chaotic household with few boundaries. Courtney attended the after-school club daily and was then left to play outside unsupervised. In contrast to the school's picture of a sexually precocious pre-adolescent, we saw a needy toddler. Courtney refused to go to bed, demanded baths at midnight, helped herself to food at all hours and was put to sleep in her parents' bed with a bottle. 'She'll drive you to drink!' joked the father, 'I just want to kill *it* sometimes', said her mother.

Courtney's parents seemed like needy children themselves. It felt imperative to offer them regular support, and to mend the mutually blaming relationship between family and school.

When individual sessions started with my colleague Becky some weeks later, Courtney's behaviour was increasingly violent, 'attacking' staff and 'trashing' rooms. She was frequently excluded, the staff room groaning at the very mention of her name. The little girl who cried so often for her mother became, in their minds, a threatening dangerous figure. Becky, on meeting Courtney, felt surprised; although tall for her age and chunky, she was, after all, a 7-year-old child. Becky wrote:

> *In early sessions I felt plunged into a chaotic, deprived world. She stripped dolls of clothes with her teeth, climbed on furniture, poured water on the floor and begged for new toys. I often felt cruelly withholding. Courtney's inability to say hello or goodbye indicated powerful feelings aroused by separations and re-unions. I quickly rethought addressing her in the first person – 'I wonder if you're feeling ...' as Courtney clearly could not tolerate feeling vulnerable, screaming at me to shut up, threatening me with chairs, rushing to the toilet. I began to talk in the third person, 'Becky and Courtney', finding different ways to address her vulnerable and omnipotent feelings. 'There seems to be a Big Courtney who wants to look after everything herself, and a Little Courtney who's worried about how much she's got to manage.' Such careful phrasing calmed her somewhat.*

Courtney's return after Christmas was difficult. The family had suffered another bereavement and the teacher most trusted by the parents was on extended sick leave. Courtney regularly ran off site, struggling especially with unstructured times. She begged to go home, hit fellow pupils and attacked staff who tried to restrain her. Her parents had weekly sessions and professionals across agencies regularly convened. We liaised weekly with Courtney's teacher and support staff, trying to keep sympathy for her alive within a punitive system, working with staff to understand the impact of her traumatic past and chaotic family. In one session after a break Becky reported:

> *I went to collect Courtney from her classroom. She glanced up, looking fleetingly worried. I smiled at her and waited. My entrance into the classroom often provoked her, so I decided to wait by the door, aware of my anxiety. Soon Courtney folded her arms in an exaggerated fashion and scowled. The classroom felt still, the children staring, quiet with anticipation. I smiled again at Courtney and said 'Hello'. She dropped her eyes, shuffled around me and bolted out, slamming the door behind her. As I followed, I tried hard to imagine how the break would replicate her feelings of rejection, how she might need to project rejection into me. I passed a support teacher who rolled her eyes. My confidence was sinking. I opened the door with a dejected feeling. Courtney stood with her back to me, muttering furiously about wanting a friend with her. 'It's not fair is it?' I grumbled in pretend crossness, desperately trying to reflect what I thought Courtney was feeling, hoping that her feeling she was understood might stop another huge enactment. She swung round, shrieking 'Leave me alone.' 'You're furious!' I replied, echoing her tone, trying to show that I understood her feelings. Her scowl faded, she eyed me with curiosity and made her way to the piano. She kicked off her shoes, saying brightly, 'Pretend you're the mummy babysitting and I'm the big sister doing homework.'*

Becky had borne the onslaught, not retaliated or become punitive. Courtney became interested in attempts to understand her, responding positively to her 'baby' feelings being looked after. Yet teachers experienced Courtney's behaviour as an affront, arguing that she 'should know better', losing sight of the fragile Courtney. The little girl we saw contrasted starkly with the formidable presence that rampaged through the collective mind of staff. Calls to exclude her were renewed, a fantasy that without Courtney the school could return to working order.

The relationship between school and family became increasingly strained with this threat of exclusion. The parents again felt abandoned by the school. We called a meeting attended by the parents, social worker and head teacher, the school's reading specialist, the local authority inclusion service and ourselves. This provided a containing space to think about the emotional complexity of the case. The impact was almost immediate, Courtney managed a full week in school, her parents attended their sessions again and the school invited us to contribute to their application for extra support. When we worked together, splitting and projection abated and the situation calmed. As often happens, when grown-ups feel contained, the child relaxes and behaviour improves.

Courtney could increasingly stay in the room for whole sessions. She was building trust and confidence, both in her therapist and her place in school. She could better manage separations, and some painful feelings.

> *'Pretend this is my babe', said Courtney, holding up a doll, 'and she has to go to hospital for three weeks.'*
>
> *'Goodness', Becky replied, 'Three weeks, that does seem like a long time.' Courtney nodded seriously. 'And we didn't see each other for three weeks because of the Easter break, I wonder what that felt like?'*
>
> *'Actually, I checked on the computer', replied Courtney, 'and it was 16 weeks!'*
>
> *'It probably felt like you were left for ages', Becky said. Courtney hurled the doll across the room, 'Pretend you're my servant', she barked, 'Clear up this mess!'*

Courtney was closer to tolerating her neediness, which also helped her manage other aspects of school life. After the summer break, she seemed to have retained hopeful feelings about the therapy. The work with her parents re-started while we established links with her new teacher and support staff. This extract is from near the next half-term. She was playing at being an 'extremely rich lady'!

> *'Holiday', snapped Courtney, 'Yes, I'll go on holiday. I don't have anyone to go with, but I can buy anything I want.' She strutted around the room picking up and tossing away various 'expensive'*

objects – sunglasses, a silk scarf, trying to cope with the painful feelings of Becky going away (at half term) by being the one swanning off on holiday.

'I think Courtney really needs to know that Becky will be back after the holidays and that she'll be thinking of her.'

'Shut up', barked Courtney crossly, without looking at Becky.

'Oh, that Becky's talking again', Becky replied.

'And no one's listening', Courtney snapped as she re-arranged the covers on the doll cradle. She could not have tolerated this exchange even months before, would probably have run out of the room. Becky wondered aloud about the feeling of being shut out over the break, 'I think Courtney really wants me to know what it feels like to be excluded.' She stood up, marched towards Becky, opened her make-believe door and pretended to slap her fiercely across the face. 'I think Courtney is showing me really angry, hurting feelings and needs to know that Becky is strong enough to look after all her feelings.'

Courtney pretended to use a telephone. 'Can you come and look after the baby?' she asked 'I'm going out.' She was now more able to accept the baby parts of herself, and Becky noted aloud how Courtney now believed that Becky could look after the littler Courtney. She climbed on to the bed, pulling a blanket over her, impressively staying in touch with fragile feelings.

'Some children have sad feelings when Becky goes away', Becky said tentatively. Courtney, looked up with interest. 'It's unbelievable that Becky will be back after the holiday', Becky continued. Courtney emerged from the covers and began doing cartwheels and somersaults. 'Courtney is suddenly very energetic and full of life.' Becky noted. 'Watch this one', Courtney called, clearly full of confidence, trust and hope, at least momentarily.

In the next period we witnessed her growing ability to tolerate the painful feelings stirred up by separations. Where she had once bolted or screamed 'Shut up!' she now said, 'Ssh, I know, it's half term.' She became able to say 'hello' and sometimes even 'goodbye'. Her teacher commented on her new emotional language and her parents joked that she 'counselled' them at home. She had developed an expectation of being in her therapist's and the staffs' minds. The chaos of the outside world was intruding less dramatically on her mind and therapy. She enacted games in which she was a destitute orphan or a wartime evacuee, allowing a place to process her acute sense of deprivation.

Much energy was expended informally liaising with staff. The service's visibility and availability was vital, allowing informal conversations with the learning mentor, catch-up time with her teacher, helping staff to keep Courtney's vulnerability in mind. This lessened the anxieties felt by staff in relation to her. While her session material remained confidential, conversations with staff could helpfully convey some understanding of Courtney's mind and motivations. Her parents were appreciative of our presence, using us as a helpful link between them and the school. When tensions ran high, they made use of informal encounters, often outside the head teacher's office or in the school foyer, these generally bringing down the emotional temperature.

Sadly, Becky soon had to leave the service. Courtney's progress is evident in these moments from her last session, as she struggled, bravely, to process the feelings evoked by the ending.

She took plasticine from the tray, popped it into her mouth and began to chew. It was a bleak sight. She chewed with neither a flinch nor a grimace. Becky wondered whether Courtney did not know what she would feed on after therapy. Courtney spat out the plasticine, took paper from her box and drew squiggly pretend writing as she said, 'Dear Becky. Class 6 really wants you to come back, you were a brilliant helper and we miss you, love class 6.' Becky felt deeply touched, acknowledging that Courtney really wanted her to know how much she would miss her. 'Not me', she said quickly, 'Class 6'. 'Oh yes', Becky replied, 'Class 6'. She handed Becky a piece of paper. 'You have to write back now', she said, 'Go on!' Becky hesitated, uncertain what to do, but began to write. 'Thank you for your letter. I cannot stay but I know that you want to thank me for my help and that you will miss me. I will be thinking of you a lot and hoping things go really well.' Courtney listened, at first looking pleased, but then said, 'You're supposed to say yes . . . ' with a bewildered look. She gritted her teeth and ripped the letter down the middle.

The ending was a little too painful to process. However, the good work continued, both in school and outside. The parents were met with for long while, and four years later we learnt that, despite ups and downs, she had been held within the school until her transfer to a mainstream secondary school. By a happy coincidence her new school also had a CAMHS service that I managed, and she was offered further therapeutic work. The more vulnerable children and families often need extra help at specific times, particularly around major transitions.

Courtney gained something important with her from her therapy, yet the individual work would have been ineffective without engaging parents, teachers and other professionals. Individual therapy alone would probably have led to Courtney becoming another scapegoat excluded from the school. Instead she had experienced feeling understood, being seen not just as bad, but as hurting, as confused, responding to her circumstances. It requires painstaking effort to help staff bear the feelings that such children stir up in us. When it goes well, this can lead to change in the whole school culture. Both the referred child and other children can be thought about differently, with less reactivity and more compassion. Focusing on the system as well as individual children creates a thoughtful, less judgemental space, minimising splitting and projection, leading to less brittle psychic structures, both in the child, and in the institution.

Concluding thoughts

Anton Obholzer (Obholzer et al., 2003) suggested that educational institutions carry hopes that our children will be equipped to live in the society of the future. School staff are deeply committed to this, but, when faced with challenging behaviour, can feel that their commitment is spat back in their faces. Then despondency can set in, even a retaliatory rage.

Work in schools is subtle and difficult, hence there are good grounds for employing experienced therapists for such work. Often the cases are especially complex cases, ones that never make it to clinics. It is challenging to apply clinical skills, honed primarily on consulting rooms, to the less safe setting of a school, without the security afforded by normal therapeutic frames. A school-based therapy service should offer an array of interventions, from individual work, detailed observations of children, work with families, parents, staff and networks, trainings in psychological development, therapeutic groups and much else that requires experience, skill and authority.

The task is somewhat akin to working in a therapeutic community. One never knows when one is doing therapeutic work, when one is on or off duty, as therapy does not begin and end in sessions. In multi-agency meetings we need to monitor the anxieties flying around, and think carefully about how we deport ourselves, neither too 'stand-offish' and therapist-like, nor too involved and concrete. We are not fully part of the school system, and yet cannot be too far outside it either.

Children often stir up powerful emotions in the adults around them, of uselessness, rage, fear, hurt, which can lead to a culture of blaming and splitting. Part of our job is to disrupt this cycle of blame, by helping to understand the meaning of children's behaviour and contain the complex feelings evoked, which in turn can provide relief and diminish acting-out cycles. We hope that children who might otherwise be viewed as unwelcome presences can find a home in the institution, in the minds of the adults who care for them and hopefully feel more at home in themselves, in their own skins, which can enable them to take their place in society. In such work, and generally in therapy, we aim to create a safe external and internal 'dwelling place' for clients, colleagues and ourselves, to combat the sense of being 'disarticulated from personal belonging' (Cooper and Lousada, 2005).

Chapter 14

Concluding thoughts

This chapter provides some final thoughts about the book's central themes. I have described a personal odyssey into the lives of children and young people, and tried to distil key features of what I believe leads to emotional change and growth. To oversimplify, the root of change, I believe, lies in compassionate, thoughtful relationships, both with others, and with ourselves. It feels a privilege to accompany such an astonishing array of characters on parts of their life journeys, particularly in cases where we see profound shifts into new ways of being, thinking and feeling, new embodied stances, new relational possibilities.

Such shifts towards emotional health are generally slow and incremental, always both backward and forwards, but never without hopeful developments. Sometimes the most profound change is in learning to accept what is, rather than ceaselessly struggle to escape one's predicament. This of course has been called 'radical acceptance', knowing what we can change, accepting what we cannot and 'the wisdom to know the difference'.

We are inevitably personally touched by those we work with. Underneath our veneers we are emotional, passionate human beings. Many of us, myself certainly included, are full of peculiar foibles, odd neuroses and unfathomable contradictions. Accepting these in ourselves enables us to be more open and compassionate to similar traits in others, allowing ourselves and those we work with to experience life more fully, remaining emotionally open to whatever life throws at us.

I know I am not alone in feeling an excruciating pang of loss for people I once worked with, with whom I have had deep relational encounters. Even though they remain alive in my mind, and I know they generally have internalised something important that they carry within them, I am human enough to feel sad about not knowing what happened to them as their lives unfolded.

I do not wish to be sentimental. Every ending has losses but also gains, including relief at the end to the intensity and emotional challenges that such meetings can evoke, as Winnicott described beautifully in his paper 'Hate in the Countertransference' (1953). Nonetheless, even in my least successful cases, something has always been learnt and gained, if often painfully.

As the book ends, I again find myself wondering what inhibited or facilitated the processes whereby the characters who people these pages grew and developed. I have described the specifics in some detail, for example that neglected children need help to become more enlivened, dysregulated children to feel calm and ease. I have described the importance of managing mismatches and rebounding from them, how we must be able to bear being attacked and denigrated and also bear being loved. I have shown how often with trauma sufferers we need to build a sense of the ordinary, the hopeful, before we can tackle the actual trauma, and how with violent and abusive people, we must walk the tightrope between being in touch with both the victim and perpetrator in them.

While such technical details are I hope described in the foregoing pages, there is also something more personal to think about, the question of what is it that we must tap into if we are to successfully reach out to others in a way that gives rise to emotional growth.

At the centre of this book has been the conviction that it is the quality of relationships, of in-depth meetings, which make the difference. As much therapy research has shown (Wampold and Wampold, 2015) the therapeutic alliance is as predictive as just about anything of whether a therapy is successful. I have tried to unpick key aspects of how such an alliance manifests in moment-by-moment intersubjective encounters. Central has been the lesson described in early chapters, of needing to have one foot in and one out of the ditch. We must be able to really join with those we work with in their distress yet also not get lost with them in their ditches.

Neither being too emotionally resonant nor too emotionally distant is important. Compassion is very different to overly resonant empathy (Singer and Klimecki, 2014), which can lead to burnout and empathic distress in the practitioner and is not helpful to the recipient. It is though helpful to genuinely hope for the best for the other, while not being overly invested in the outcome. This means being sufficiently emotionally resonant to know deeply what the other is feeling (one foot in the ditch), to feel 'with' them, while simultaneously planting the other foot firmly outside the ditch, where we can reflect on, metabolise and process the experiences. At best we reach out to the other from a place of genuine care, while in part remaining on a solid bank with good footings, neither too detached nor close.

Often it is either powerful projections, or our personal issues and blocks, which inhibit genuine connection with another. For me, this means struggling to feel compassion for personality traits that I find hard to like, in myself or others. Inevitably other people trigger personal issues.

Take Molly, who appeared in the first two chapters, the semi-autistic and depressed little girl who eventually came vibrantly to life. It was easy for me to feel empathy for her fearfulness and lack of confidence. I knew about this well from my own shaky early childhood, my low self-esteem, my fear of others, traits about which, after years of therapy, I had learnt to feel more self-compassion. Probably as a 20-year-old, before my personal therapy, I might have been as frustrated and impatient with those aspects of her as I then was with myself.

Her depression was a bigger challenge, the way her wobbly equanimity could give way to searing despair from which almost nothing seemed able to rescue her. Her deep dark desolation needed to be tolerated in order for me to really help her. I needed to have faith, in myself, that such despairing depression could be both borne, stayed with, and recovered from, that there can be light at the end of such dark tunnels. Only then could I really reach out to her experience, and help her.

By the same token, I needed to know enough about exuberance, joy, becoming assertive and agentic to help her experience really positive emotions. It was no coincidence that initially I mistakenly empathised with hurt toy animals that she repaired by putting plasters on them, representing her belief in a fragile and damaged internal world, rather than a robust one. I needed the enlivening presence of my brilliant supervisor, Anne Alvarez, but also to have ventured out of inhibited fearfulness in myself into a more courageous life stance, to really help

Molly. I will never forget how difficult it was initially to join her exuberantly, as we flung toys across the room, but how liberating it was when we did so.

Much gets in the way of reaching out and genuinely being with another. For those of us who honed empathy skills in somewhat dysfunctional families, a big issue is having too great a need to look after the other, being too attached to making others feel better. This is part of what Bion (1967) described as having too much 'memory and desire', what many in contemplative traditions warn of as being too attached to outcomes. This has multiple dangers, including becoming burnt out. We can feel hurt, despondent, rejected or inadequate when our 'kind care' is not accepted. Most importantly, no one wants to feel pressured to change to make someone else feel better. Being with another, genuinely wanting the best for them, but not being overly attached to a specific outcome, is an important state of mind to cultivate. I find I am particularly helped in this by my mindfulness practice, as well as good colleagues and supervision.

It is all too easy to retreat to a professional defensiveness, seeing problems and psychopathologies as residing in the other, but not in ourselves. Condescension never feels good to be on the receiving end of. We all have our own versions of denial. Working with violent young people, for example, I can easily assume that I am not capable of the heinous acts they perpetrate. We all prefer to think that 'we' are incapable of such deeds, just as we all think that if we were born in Nazi Germany we would have been the rare morally courageous ones. The Milgram experiments (Milgram, 1974), among others, should leave us in no doubt how we can deceive ourselves.

Dillon, mentioned in Chapter 12, had powerful paedophilic drives, and this challenged my own sense of morality and what I could tolerate, as well as my capacity for empathy. Work with forensic patients can only succeed if we can reach out to both the perpetrator and the victim in them, not shirk their psychic realities, but somehow retain compassion for their predicaments.

We all have angry, even murderous feelings, whether to siblings, rivals in love, career competitors, or those who have wronged us. It is only by making friends with such parts of ourselves, befriending or 'taming' feelings like hatred, envy, rage or despair, that, we can really help others. People stuck deep in ditches need to know that we too understand what it is like down there, that we can bear feeling feelings like theirs, but also that we know that such feelings do not define us. Psychoanalysis like mindfulness helps us to stay with and make friends with what we are naturally averse to.

Some of my most difficult cases have featured neglect, as I wrote about earlier. Most of us are challenged by the deadness, cut-offness and lack of interpersonal ease we encounter when working with highly neglected children. We are an emotionally resonant species and don't like to resonate with dullness, or be treated as less than human. Yet to work with such patients I needed to know something of my own deadened traits, the parts of me that can shut down when threatened, the baby I once was who was left alone with strangers for long periods, the 9-year-old sent to boarding school, the adolescent who no one 'got'. This was a me who had to fend for himself, who managed by retreating into semi-dissociative states and repetitive activities and nearly gave up on lively passionate relationships. Now I feel I understand, indeed love, the little boy I once was, and that has helped me reach out to cut-off children I have worked with.

This is not the version of me I like to present to the world. I prefer people to see the boy who eventually became popular and liked in school, who was talented at athletics, felt brilliant at football, was clever in many subjects, developed a good sense of humour, was caring and passionate. That is all me too, but I still have a tendency to become like neglected patients who retreat. That is the me who can spend too long on my computer, who might obsessionally perseverate, who can be a touch too organised. It is only in learning to accept, indeed love those parts of ourselves that we can offer out our whole beings to people in similar ditches.

These personal revelations are made for a reason. We of course must be well trained to do this work, to understand the issues that people present with, and know what can help. Without this we can fail people, as I demonstrated in my unhelpful early work with traumatised dissociated people before I understood what they require.

We also need good supervision, colleagues we can rely on and an ability to stay open, curious, indeed passionate about, our work. We certainly also need a rich enough life outside the consulting room.

Personally, I could not do this work without undergoing my own personal psychotherapy and analysis, each over many years, often many times a week. I also could not do this work without an ongoing set of personal practices, which for me are primarily sitting daily on my mindfulness stool, regular yoga, the gym and the blissful solitude of running. Yet it is in interpersonal, intimate human encounters where we are most challenged to grow and that more than anything re-fuel and safeguard an openness to life. This pays unquantifiable dividends in the consulting room.

To do this work, we must open to the darkest and most difficult parts of ourselves, the parts we would rather deny, ignore or project into others. This in effect means joining ourselves too in whatever ditches we are prone to fall deeply into. It means having the kind of relationship with ourselves that is also the kind that is at the root of successful therapy, a generous, self-compassionate but unflinchingly honest relationship, a therapeutic alliance with ourselves as well as others.

Therapeutic protocols, techniques, methodologies and schools of thought can be helpful, even essential, but are never enough. Manuals can suggest effective techniques but not how to become open-hearted courageous people capable of meeting others in their depths. Rather, we need to grope in the dark, get lost, be uncertain, take risks, be honest, face the most difficult aspects of ourselves and others, as well as the most hopeful. Genuinely meeting another can never be about techniques or skills. It must be about being a feeling-full, flawed, but emotionally open, full-blooded human being, however that is defined. It is our relationships, with ourselves and others that in the end are curative. This is not easy to hold on to in our world of manualised treatments, national guidelines, commissioning priorities and black and white ideas. Such a commitment to compassionate relationships, with others and ourselves, is vitally needed, I believe, for our clients, ourselves and for humanity's future.

Bibliography

Alvarez, A. (1992) *Live Company*. London: Routledge.

Alvarez, A. (1995) Motiveless malignity: Problems in the psychotherapy of psychopathic patients, *Journal of Child Psychotherapy*, 21 (2), pp. 167–182.

Alvarez, A. (2012) *The Thinking Heart: Three Levels of Psychoanalytic Therapy with Disturbed Children*. Oxford: Routledge.

Armstrong, D. and Rustin, M. (eds) (2014) *Social Defences against Anxiety: Explorations in a Paradigm*. London: Karnac.

Aron, L. (2001) *A Meeting of Minds: Mutuality in Psychoanalysis*. New York: Analytic Press.

Arsenio, W. F. and Gold, J. (2006) The effects of social injustice and inequality on children's moral judgments and behavior: Towards a theoretical model, *Cognitive Development*, 21 (4), pp. 388–400.

Bakermans-Kranenburg, M. J. and van IJzendoorn, M. H. (2015) The hidden efficacy of interventions: Gene × environment experiments from a differential susceptibility perspective, *Annual Review of Psychology*, 66 (1), pp. 381–409.

Balint, M. (1968) *The Basic Fault: Therapeutic Aspects of Regression*. London: Tavistock.

Barkley, R. A. (2012) *Executive Functions: What They Are, How They Work, and Why They Evolved*. New York: Guilford Press.

Bateson, M. C. (1971) The interpersonal context of infant vocalization, *Quarterly Progress Report of the Research Laboratory of Electronics*, 100, pp. 170–176.

Beebe, B., Knoblauch, S., Rustin, J., Sorter, D., Jacobs, T. J. and Pally, R. (2005) *Forms of Intersubjectivity in Infant Research and Adult Treatment*. New York: Other Press.

Beebe, B. and Lachmann, F. M. (2002) *Infant Research and Adult Treatment: Co-Constructing Interactions*. New York: Analytic Press.

Bekhterev, V. M. (1907) *Objective Psychology*. St. Petersburg: Soikin.

Benjamin, J. (1998) *Like Subjects, Love Objects: Essays on Recognition and Sexual Difference*. New Haven, CT: Yale University Press.

Bhanji, J. P. and Delgado, M. R. (2014) The social brain and reward: Social information processing in the human striatum, *Wiley Interdisciplinary Reviews: Cognitive Science*, 5 (1), pp. 61–73.

Bick, E. (1968) The experience of the skin in early object relations, *International Journal of Psycho-Analysis*, 49, pp. 484–486.

Bion, W. R. (1962a) A theory of thinking, *Melanie Klein Today: Developments in Theory and Practice*, 1, pp. 178–186.

Bion, W. R. (1962b) *Learning from Experience*. London: Heinemann.

Bion, W. R. (1967) Notes on memory and desire, *Psychoanalytic Forum*, 2 (3), pp. 271–280.

Bion, W. R. (2013) *Attention and Interpretation: A Scientific Approach to Insight in Psycho-Analysis and Groups*. Oxford: Routledge.

Bisby, M. A., Kimonis, E. R. and Goulter, N. (2017) Low maternal warmth mediates the relationship between emotional neglect and callous-unemotional traits among male juvenile offenders, *Journal of Child and Family Studies*, 26 (7), pp. 1790–1798.

Bischof-Köhler, D. (2012) Empathy and self-recognition in phylogenetic and ontogenetic perspective, *Emotion Review*, 4 (1), pp. 40–48.

Bjorklund, D. F. (2007) *Why Youth Is Not Wasted on the Young: Immaturity in Human Development*. Oxford: Blackwell.

Blair, R. J. R. (2018) Traits of empathy and anger: Implications for psychopathy and other disorders associated with aggression, *Philosophical Transactions of the Royal Society B*, 373, p. 1744. doi: 10.1098/rstb.2017.0155.

Bogdan, R. and Pizzagalli, D. A. (2006) Acute stress reduces reward responsiveness: Implications for depression, *Biological Psychiatry*, 60 (10), pp. 1147–1154.

Bollas, C. (1987) *The Shadow of the Object: Psychoanalysis of the Unthought Known*. London: Free Association Books.

Bollas, C. (1989) *Forces of Destiny: Psychoanalysis and Human Idiom*. London: Free Association Books.

Borelli, J. L., Ho, L. C., Sohn, L., Epps, L., Coyiuto, M. and West, J. L. (2016) School-aged children's attachment dismissal prospectively predicts divergence of their behavioral and self-reported anxiety, *Journal of Child and Family Studies*, 26, pp. 1018–1026.

Bos, P. A. (2017) The endocrinology of human caregiving and its intergenerational transmission, *Development and Psychopathology*, 29 (3), pp. 971–999.

Boston Process of Change Group. (2010) *Change in Psychotherapy: A Unifying Paradigm*. New York: W.W. Norton & Company.

Bowlby, J. (1969) *Attachment and Loss. Vol. 1, Attachment*. London: Hogarth.

Brand, M., Snagowski, J., Laier, C. and Maderwald, S. (2016) Ventral striatum activity when watching preferred pornographic pictures is correlated with symptoms of internet pornography addiction, *NeuroImage*, 129, pp. 224–232.

Bråten, S. (1998) *Intersubjective Communication and Emotion in Early Ontogeny*. Cambridge: Cambridge University Press.

Brazelton, T. B. and Cramer, B. G. (1991) *The Earliest Relationship: Parents, Infants, and the Drama of Early Attachment*. London: Karnac.

Britton, R., O'Shaughnessy, M. and Feldman, M. (1989) *The Oedipus Complex Today: Clinical Implications*. London: Karnac.

Bronfenbrenner, U. (2004) *Making Human Beings Human: Bioecological Perspectives on Human Development*. CA: Sage.

Calhoun, L. G. and Tedeschi, R. G. (2014) *Handbook of Posttraumatic Growth: Research and Practice*. Oxford: Routledge.

Carpenter, M., Uebel, J. and Tomasello, M. (2013) Being mimicked increases prosocial behavior in 18-month-old infants, *Child Development*, 84 (5), pp. 1511–1518.

Carr, N. (2011) *The Shallows: What the Internet Is Doing to Our Brains*. New York: Norton.

Chiesa, A., Serretti, A. and Jakobsen, J. C. (2013) Mindfulness: Top-down or bottom-up emotion regulation strategy? *Clinical Psychology Review*, 33 (1), pp. 82–96.

Cicchetti, D. (2010) Resilience under conditions of extreme stress: A multilevel perspective, *World Psychiatry*, 9 (3), pp. 145–154.

Coltart, N. (1992) *Slouching towards Bethlehem*. London: Free Association Books.

Cooper, A. and Lousada, J. (2005) *Borderline Welfare: Feeling and Fear of Feeling in Modern Welfare*. London: Karnac.

Corrigan, E. and Gordon, P.-E. (1995) *The Mind Object*. London: Karnac.

Cozolino, L. (2006) *The Neuroscience of Human Relationships: Attachment and the Developing Social Brain*. New York: W. W. Norton & Co.

Dalley, J. W. and Robbins, T. W. (2017) Fractionating impulsivity: Neuropsychiatric implications, *Nature Reviews Neuroscience*, 18 (3), pp. 158–171.

Damasio, A. R. (1999) *The Feeling of What Happens: Body, Emotion and the Making of Consciousness*. London: Heineman.

Damasio, A. R. (2012) *Self Comes to Mind: Constructing the Conscious Brain*. London: Vintage.

Davidson, R. J. (2000) Affective style, psychopathology, and resilience: Brain mechanisms and plasticity, *The American Psychologist*, 55 (11), pp. 1196–1214.

Dawkins, R. (2006) *The Selfish Gene*. Oxford: Oxford University Press.

DeJong, M. (2010) Some reflections on the use of psychiatric diagnosis in the looked after or 'in care' child population, *Clinical Child Psychology and Psychiatry*, 15 (4), pp. 589–599.

Duckworth, A. L., Quinn, P. D. and Tsukayama, E. (2011) What no child left behind leaves behind: The roles of IQ and self-control in predicting standardized achievement test scores and report card grades, *Journal of Educational Psychology*, 104 (2), pp. 439–451.

Duffell, N. (2000) *The Making of Them: The British Attitude to Children and the Boarding School System*. Bland, R. (ed.) London: Lone Arrow Press.

Eagleman, D. (2011) *Incognito: The Secret Lives of the Brain*. New York: Pantheon.

Eliot, G. (1985) *The Mill on the Floss. 1860*. Byatt, A. S. (ed.). Harmondsworth: Penguin.

Eluvathingal, T. J., Chugani, H. T., Behen, M. E., Juhasz, C., Muzik, O., Maqbool, M., Chugani, D. C. and Makki, M. (2006) Abnormal brain connectivity in children after early severe socioemotional deprivation: A diffusion tensor imaging study, *Pediatrics*, 117 (6), pp. 2093–2100.

Emanuel, L. (2002) Deprivation× 3, *Journal of Child Psychotherapy*, 28 (2), pp. 163–179.

Fairbairn, W. R. D. (1962) *An Object-Relations Theory of the Personality*. New York: Basic Books.

Farb, N., Daubenmier, J., Price, C. J., Gard, T., Kerr, C., Dunn, B. D., Klein, A. C., Paulus, M. P. and Mehling, W. E. (2015) Interoception, contemplative practice, and health, *Frontiers in Psychology*, 6 [online]. doi: 10.3389/fpsyg.2015.00763.

Field, T. (2011) Prenatal depression effects on early development: A review, *Infant Behavior and Development*, 34 (1), pp. 1–14.

Field, T., Diego, M. and Hernandez-Reif, M. (2006) Prenatal depression effects on the fetus and newborn: A review, *Infant Behavior and Development*, 29 (3), pp. 445–455.

Fonagy, P. and Allison, E. (2014) The role of mentalizing and epistemic trust in the therapeutic relationship, *Psychotherapy*, 51 (3), pp. 372–380.

Fonagy, P., Gyorgy, G., Jurist, E. L. and Target, M. (2004) *Affect Regulation, Mentalization, and the Development of the Self*. London: Karnac.

Fonagy, P., Target, M., Cottrell, D., Phillips, J. and Kurtz, Z. (2005) *What Works for Whom? A Critical Review of Treatments for Children and Adolescents*. New York: Guilford.

Ford, T., Vostanis, P., Meltzer, H. and Goodman, R. (2007) Psychiatric disorder among British children looked after by local authorities: Comparison with children living in private households, *British Journal of Psychiatry*, 190 (4), pp. 319–325.

Foucault, M. (2002) *Power: The Essential Works of Michel Foucault 1954–1984* (3rd ed.). London: Penguin.

Fraiberg, S. (1974) Blind infants and their mothers: An examination of the sign system, in: Lewis, M. and Rosenblum, L. A. (eds) *The Effect of the Infant on Its Caregiver*. Oxford: Wiley, pp. 215–232.

Freud, S. (1920/2001) Beyond the pleasure principle, in: Strachey, J. (ed.) *The Standard Edition of the Complete Psychological Works of Sigmund Freud*. London: Vintage, p. 18.

Fumero, A., Marrero, R. J., Voltes, D. and Peñate, W. (2018) Personal and social factors involved in internet addiction among adolescents: A meta-analysis, *Computers in Human Behavior*, 86, pp. 387–400. doi: 10.1016/j.chb.2018.05.005.

Gazzaniga, M. S. (2006) *The Ethical Brain: The Science of Our Moral Dilemmas*. New York: Harper.

Gelso, C. J. (2010) *The Real Relationship in Psychotherapy: The Hidden Foundation of Chance*. Washington, DC: American Psychological Association.

Gentile, D. A., Swing, E. L., Lim, C. G. and Khoo, A. (2012) Video game playing, attention problems, and impulsiveness: Evidence of bidirectional causality, *Psychology of Popular Media Culture*, 1 (1), pp. 62–70.

Gilbert, P. (2014) The origins and nature of compassion-focused therapy, *British Journal of Clinical Psychology*, 53 (1), pp. 6–41.

Gilligan, J. (2009) Sex, gender and violence: Estela Welldon's contribution to our understanding of the psychopathology of violence, *British Journal of Psychotherapy*, 25 (2), pp. 239–256.

Glasser, M. (1986) Identification and its vicissitudes as observed in the perversions, *International Journal of Psychoanalysis*, 67 (1), pp. 9–17.

Glasser, M. (1992) Problems in the psychoanalysis of certain narcissistic disorders, *International Journal of Psychoanalysis*, 73 (3), pp. 493–503.

Goleman, D. (2006) *Emotional Intelligence*. New York: Bantam.

Gordon, P. (1999) *Face to Face: Therapy as Ethics*. London: Constable.

Graf, D. L., Pratt, L. V., Hester, C. N. and Short, K. R. (2009) Playing active video games increases energy expenditure in children, *Pediatrics*, 124 (2), pp. 534–540.

Graziano, P. and Derefinko, K. (2013) Cardiac vagal control and children's adaptive functioning: A meta-analysis, *Biological Psychology*, 94 (1), pp. 22–37.

Greenspan, S. I. and Downey, J. I. (1997) *Developmentally Based Psychotherapy*. Madison, WI: International Universities Press.

Griffiths, M. D., Kuss, D. J. and Ortiz de Gortari, A. B. (2017) Video games as therapy: An updated selective review of the medical and psychological literature,

International Journal of Privacy and Health Information Management, 5 (2), pp. 71–96.

Grubbs, J. B., Stauner, N., Exline, J. J., Pargament, K. I. and Lindberg, M. J. (2015) Perceived addiction to internet pornography and psychological distress: Examining relationships concurrently and over time, *Psychology of Addictive Behaviors*, 29 (4), pp. 1056–1067.

Gullhaugen, A. S. and Nøttestad, J. A. (2012) Under the surface the dynamic interpersonal and affective world of psychopathic high-security and detention prisoners, *International Journal of Offender Therapy and Comparative Criminology*, 56 (6), pp. 917–936.

Guntrip, H. (1995) *Schizoid Phenomena, Object Relations and the Self*. London: Karnac.

Hafiz. (1999) *The Gift: Poems by Hafiz the Great Sufi Master*. New York: Penguin Books.

Haglund, M. E. M., Nestadt, P. S., Cooper, N. S., Southwick, S. M. and Charney, D. S. (2007) Psychobiological mechanisms of resilience: Relevance to prevention and treatment of stress-related psychopathology, *Development and Psychopathology*, 19 (3), pp. 889–920.

Hamlin, J. K., Wynn, K. and Bloom, P. (2007) Social evaluation by preverbal infants, *Nature*, 450 (7169), pp. 557–559.

Hatfield, E., Cacioppo, J. T. and Rapson, R. L. (1993) Emotional contagion, *Current Directions in Psychological Science*, 2 (3), pp. 96–99.

Hazell, J. (1996) *H.J.S. Guntrip: A Psychoanalytical Biography*. London; New York: Free Association Books.

Heller, M. and Haynal, V. (1997) The doctor's face: A mirror of his patient's suicidal projects, in: Guimón, J. (ed.) *The Body in Psychotherapy*. Basel, Switzerland: Karger, pp. 46–51.

Henry, G. (1974) Doubly deprived, *Journal of Child Psychotherapy*, 3 (4), pp. 15–28.

Hobson, R. P. and Lee, A. (1989) Emotion-related and abstract concepts in autistic people: Evidence from the British picture vocabulary scale, *Journal of Autism and Developmental Disorders*, 19 (4), pp. 601–623.

Holmes, J. and Slade, A. (2017) *Attachment in Therapeutic Practice*. Thousand Oaks, CA: Sage.

Hughes, D. A. (2007) *Attachment-Focused Family Therapy*. New York: Norton.

Jackson, E. (2008) The development of work discussion groups in educational settings, *Journal of Child Psychotherapy*, 34 (1), pp. 62–82.

Jankowski, K. F. and Takahashi, H. (2014) Cognitive neuroscience of social emotions and implications for psychopathology: Examining embarrassment, guilt, envy, and schadenfreude, *Psychiatry and Clinical Neurosciences*, 68 (5), pp. 319–336.

Jessen, S. and Grossmann, T. (2014) Unconscious discrimination of social cues from eye whites in infants, *Proceedings of the National Academy of Sciences*, 111 (45), pp. 16208–16213.

Johnson, S. C., Dweck, C. S. and Chen, F. S. (2007) Evidence for infants' internal working models of attachment, *Psychological Science*, 18 (6), pp. 501–502.

Joyce, J. (1914/1992) *Dubliners*. Harmondsworth: Penguin.

Kalivas, P. W. and Volkow, N. D. (2014) The neural basis of addiction: A pathology of motivation and choice, *American Journal of Psychiatry*, 162 (8), pp. 1403–1413.

Kasser, T. (2003) *The High Price of Materialism*. Cambridge, MA: MIT Press.

Keats, J. (1899) *The Complete Poetical Works and Letters of John Keats*. Scudder, H. E. (ed.). Boston, MA: Riverside Press.

Keleman, S. (1975) *Your Body Speaks Its Mind: The Bio-Energetic Way to Greater Emotional and Sexual Satisfaction*. New York: Simon & Schuster.

Kidd, D., Ongis, M. and Castano, E. (2016) On literary fiction and its effects on theory of mind, *Scientific Study of Literature*, 6 (1), pp. 42–58.

Kimonis, E. R., Centifanti, L. C., Allen, J. L. and Frick, P. J. (2014) Reciprocal influences between negative life events and callous-unemotional traits, *Journal of Abnormal Child Psychology*, 42 (8), pp. 1287–1298.

Klein, M. (1946) Notes on some schizoid mechanisms, *International Journal of Psycho-Analysis*, 27, pp. 99–110.

Klein, M. (1975) *The Psycho-Analysis of Children*. New York: Delacorte Press.

Knibbs, C. (2016) *Cybertrauma: The Darker Side of the Internet for Children and Young People*. Cybertrauma Works. [online].

Kochanska, G. and Kim, S. (2012) Toward a new understanding of legacy of early attachments for future antisocial trajectories: Evidence from two longitudinal studies, *Development and Psychopathology*, 1 (1), pp. 1–24.

Koole, S. L. and Tschacher, W. (2016) Synchrony in psychotherapy: A review and an integrative framework for the therapeutic alliance, *Frontiers in Psychology*, 7 [online]. doi: 10.3389/fpsyg.2016.00862.

Kowalski, R. M., Giumetti, G. W., Schroeder, A. N. and Lattanner, M. R. (2014) Bullying in the digital age: A critical review and meta-analysis of cyberbullying research among youth, *Psychological Bulletin*, 4, pp. 1073–1137.

Kraus, S. W., Voon, V. and Potenza, M. N. (2016) Neurobiology of compulsive sexual behavior: Emerging science, *Neuropsychopharmacology*, 41 (1), pp. 385–386.

Krause, A. L., Borchardt, V., Li, M., van Tol, M.-J., Demenescu, L. R. and Strauss, B., Kirchmann, H., Buchheim, A., Metzger, C. D., Nolte, T. and

Walter, M. (2016) Dismissing attachment characteristics dynamically modulate brain networks subserving social aversion, *Frontiers in Human Neuroscience*, 10 [online]. doi: 10.3389/fnhum.2016.00077.

Kuhlmeier, V., Wynn, K. and Bloom, P. (2003) Attribution of dispositional states by 12-month-olds, *Psychological Science*, 14 (5), pp. 402–408.

Kujawa, A., Wu, M., Klumpp, H., Pine, D. S., Swain, J. E., Fitzgerald, K. D., Monk, C. S. and Phan, K. L. (2016) Altered development of amygdala-anterior cingulate cortex connectivity in anxious youth and young adults, *Biological Psychiatry: Cognitive Neuroscience and Neuroimaging*, 1 (4), pp. 345–352.

Kungl, M. T., Leyh, R. and Spangler, G. (2016) Attachment representations and brain asymmetry during the processing of autobiographical emotional memories in late adolescence, *Frontiers in Human Neuroscience*, 10 [online]. doi: 10.3389/fnhum.2016.00644.

LaFrance, M. (1979) Nonverbal synchrony and rapport: Analysis by the cross-lag panel technique, *Social Psychology Quarterly*, 42, pp. 66–70.

Lambert, M. J. (2005) Early response in psychotherapy: Further evidence for the importance of common factors rather than 'placebo effects', *Journal of Clinical Psychology*, 61 (7), pp. 855–869.

Lee, Y.-K., Chang, C.-T., Cheng, Z.-H. and Lin, Y. (2018) How social anxiety and reduced self-efficacy induce smartphone addiction in materialistic people, *Social Science Computer Review*, 36 (1), pp. 36–56.

Leff, J., Williams, G., Huckvale, M., Arbuthnot, M. and Leff, A. P. (2014) Avatar therapy for persecutory auditory hallucinations: What is it and how does it work? *Psychosis*, 6 (2), pp. 166–176.

Lilliengren, P., Falkenström, F., Sandell, R., Mothander, P. R. and Werbart, A. (2015) Secure attachment to therapist, alliance, and outcome in psychoanalytic psychotherapy with young adults, *Journal of Counseling Psychology*, 62 (1), pp. 1–13.

Lockwood, P. L., Sebastian, C. L., McCrory, E. J., Hyde, Z. H., Gu, X., De Brito, S. A. and Viding, E. (2013) Association of callous traits with reduced neural responses to others' pain in children with conduct problems, *Current Biology*, 23 (10), pp. 901–905.

Lowen, A. (1975) *Bioenergetics*. New York: Coward, McCann & Geoghegan.

Luria, A. R. (1966) *Higher Cortical Functions in Man*. New York: Basic Books.

Lyons, D. M., Parker, K. J., Katz, M. and Schatzberg, A. F. (2009) Developmental cascades linking stress inoculation, arousal regulation, and resilience, *Frontiers in Behavioral Neuroscience*, 3 (32) [online]. doi: 10.3389/neuro.08.032.2009.

Lyth, I. M. (1988) *Containing Anxiety in Institutions*. London: Free Association Books.

McCrory, E. J., Puetz, V., Maguire, E., Mechelli, A., Palmer, A., Gerin, M., Kelly, P., Koutoufa, I. and Viding, E. (2017) Autobiographical memory: A candidate latent vulnerability mechanism for psychiatric disorder following childhood maltreatment, *British Journal of Psychiatry*, 211 (4), pp. 216–222.

Mcdougall, J. (1992) *Plea for a Measure of Abnormality*. London: Routledge.

Mcgilchrist, I. (2010) *The Master and His Emissary: The Divided Brain and the Making of the Western World*. New Haven, CT: Yale University Press.

MacKinnon, N., Kingsbury, M., Mahedy, L., Evans, J. and Colman, I. (2018) The association between prenatal stress and externalizing symptoms in childhood: Evidence from the Avon longitudinal study of parents and children, *Biological Psychiatry*, 83 (2), pp. 100–108. doi: 10.1016/j.biopsych.2017.07.010.

McLaughlin, K. A., Sheridan, M. A., Alves, S. and Mendes, W. B. (2014) Child maltreatment and autonomic nervous system reactivity: Identifying dysregulated stress reactivity patterns by using the biopsychosocial model of challenge and threat, *Psychosomatic Medicine*, 76 (7), pp. 538–546.

McTavish, J. R., MacGregor, J. C., Wathen, C. N. and MacMillan, H. L. (2016) Children's exposure to intimate partner violence: An overview, *International Review of Psychiatry*, 28 (5), pp. 504–518.

Maddi, S. R. (2005) On hardiness and other pathways to resilience, *American Psychologist*, 60 (3), pp. 261–262.

Maheu, F. S., Dozier, M., Guyer, A. E., Mandell, D., Peloso, E., Poeth, K., Jenness, J., Lau, J. Y., Ackerman, J. P., Pine, D. S. and Ernst, M. (2010) A preliminary study of medial temporal lobe function in youths with a history of caregiver deprivation and emotional neglect, *Cognitive, Affective, and Behavioral Neuroscience*, 10 (1), pp. 34–49.

Main, M. and George, C. (1985) Responses of abused and disadvantaged toddlers to distress in agemates: A study in the day care setting. *Developmental Psychology*, 21 (3), pp. 407–412.

Malin, A. J. and Pos, A. E. (2015) The impact of early empathy on alliance building, emotional processing, and outcome during experiential treatment of depression, *Psychotherapy Research*, 25 (4), pp. 445–459.

Márquez, C., Poirier, G. L., Cordero, M. I., Larsen, M. H., Groner, A., Marquis, J., Magistretti, P. J., Trono, D. and Sandi, C. (2013) Peripuberty stress leads to abnormal aggression, altered amygdala and orbitofrontal reactivity and increased prefrontal MAOA gene expression, *Translational Psychiatry*, 3 [online]. doi: 10.1038/tp.2012.144.

Marshall, P. J., Fox, N. A. and Group, B. C. (2004) A comparison of the electroencephalogram between institutionalized and community children in Romania, *Journal of Cognitive Neuroscience*, 16 (8), pp. 1327–1338.

Meins, E. (2012) Social relationships and children's understanding of, in: Siegal, M. and Surian, L. (eds) *Access to Language and Cognitive Development.* Oxford: Oxford University Press, pp. 1134–1145.

Meins, E., Fernyhough, C., Wainwright, R., Gupta, M. D., Fradley, E. and Tuckey, M. (2002) Maternal mind-mindedness and attachment security as predictors of theory of mind understanding, *Child Development*, 73 (6), pp. 1715–1726.

Meins, E. and Russell, J. (2011) Security and symbolic play: The relation between security of attachment and executive capacity, *British Journal of Developmental Psychology*, 15 (1), pp. 63–76.

Meltzer, D. (1975) Adhesive identification, *Contemporary Psychoanalysis*, 11, pp. 289–310.

Meltzer, D. (1976/2018) Temperature and distance as technical dimensions of interpretation, in: Hahn, A. (ed.) *Sincerity and Other Works: Collected Papers of Donald Meltzer.* London: Routledge, pp. 374–386.

Meltzer, D. (2008) *The Psycho-Analytical Process.* London: Karnac.

Meltzer, D., Williams, M. H. and Trust, R. H. (1988) *The Apprehension of Beauty: The Role of Aesthetic Conflict in Development, Violence and Art.* Perthshire: Clunie Press.

Meltzoff, A. N. (1988) Infant imitation and memory: Nine-month-olds in immediate and deferred tests, *Child Development*, 59 (1), pp. 217–225.

Mikulincer, M., Shaver, P. R., Gillath, O. and Nitzberg, R. A. (2005) Attachment, caregiving, and altruism: Boosting attachment security increases compassion and helping, *Journal of Personality and Social Psychology*, 89 (5), pp. 817–839.

Milgram, S. (1974) *Obedience to Authority: An Experimental View.* London: Tavistock.

Milner, M. (1936) *A Life of One's Own.* London: Chatto & Windus.

Mischel, W. (2014) *Marshmallow Test.* New York: Little, Brown & Company.

Moffitt, T. E., Arseneault, L., Belsky, D., Dickson, N., Hancox, R. J., Harrington, H. L., Houts, R., Poulton, R., Roberts, B. W., Ross, S., Sears, M. R., Thomson, W. M. and Caspi, A. (2011) A gradient of childhood self-control predicts health, wealth, and public safety, *Proceedings of the National Academy of Sciences*, 108 (7), pp. 2693–2698.

Moll, J., Zahn, R., de Oliveira-Souza, R., Krueger, F. and Grafman, J. (2005) The neural basis of human moral cognition, *Nature Reviews Neuroscience*, 6 (10), pp. 799–809.

Morgan, S. P. (2005) Depression: Turning toward life. Mindfulness and psychotherapy, in: Christopher, K., Siegel, R. D. and Fulton, R. (eds) *Mindfulness and Psychotherapy.* New York: Guilford, pp. 130–151.

Morrison, B. (2011) *As If.* London: Granta Books.

Moyers, T. B. and Miller, W. R. (2013) Is low therapist empathy toxic? *Psychology of Addictive Behaviors*, 27 (3), pp. 878–884.

Murray, L. and Cooper, P. (1999) *Postpartum Depression and Child Development.* New York: Guilford.

Music, G. (2005) Surfacing the depths: Thoughts on imitation, resonance and growth, *Journal of Child Psychotherapy*, 31 (1), pp. 72–90.

Music, G. (2009) What has psychoanalysis got to do with happiness? Reclaiming the positive in psychoanalytic psychotherapy, *British Journal of Psychotherapy*, 25 (4), pp. 435–455.

Music, G. (2011) Trauma, helpfulness and selfishness: The effect of abuse and neglect on altruistic, moral and pro-social capacities, *Journal of Child Psychotherapy*, 37 (2), pp. 113–128.

Music, G. (2016) *Nurturing Natures: Attachment and Children's Emotional, Social and Brain Development.* London: Psychology Press.

Nathanson, A. (2016) Embracing darkness: Clinical work with adolescents and young adults addicted to sexual enactments, *Journal of Child Psychotherapy*, 43 (3), pp. 272–284.

Negash, S., Sheppard, N. V. N., Lambert, N. M. and Fincham, F. D. (2016) Trading later rewards for current pleasure: Pornography consumption and delay discounting, *Journal of Sex Research*, 53 (6), pp. 689–700.

Nelson, C. A., Westerlund, A., McDermott, J. M., Zeanah, C. H. and Fox, N. A. (2013) Emotion recognition following early psychosocial deprivation, *Development and Psychopathology*, 25 (2), pp. 517–525.

Norcross, J. C. and Karpiak, C. P. (2017) Our best selves: Defining and actualizing expertise in psychotherapy, *The Counseling Psychologist*, 45 (1), pp. 66–75.

Norcross, J. C. and Lambert, M. J. (2014) Relationship science and practice in psychotherapy: Closing commentary, *Psychotherapy*, 51 (3), p. 398.

Oakley, B., Knafo, A., Madhavan, G. and Wilson, D. (eds) (2012) *Pathological Altruism.* Oxford: Oxford University Press.

Obholzer, A. and Roberts, D. V. Z. (eds) (2003) *The Unconscious at Work: Individual and Organizational Stress in the Human Services.* Oxford: Routledge.

Oei, A. C. and Patterson, M. D. (2013) Enhancing cognition with video games: A multiple game training study, *PLoS One*, 8 (3) [online]. doi: 10.1371/journal. pone.0058546.

Ogden, P. (2006) *Trauma and the Body: A Sensorimotor Approach to Psychotherapy.* New York: W. W. Norton & Co.

Ogden, T. H. (1999) *Reverie and Interpretation: Sensing Something Human.* London: Karnac.

Ogloff, J. R., Cutajar, M. C., Mann, E., Mullen, P., Wei, F. T. Y., Hassan, H. A. B. and Yih, T. H. (2012) Child sexual abuse and subsequent offending and victimisation: A 45-year follow-up study, *Trends and Issues in Crime and Criminal Justice*, 440 (1), pp. 1836–2206.

Olds, J. and Milner, P. (1954) Positive reinforcement produced by electrical stimulation of septal area and other regions of rat brain, *Journal of Comparative and Physiological Psychology*, 47 (6), pp. 419–427.

Pakulak, E., Stevens, C. and Neville, H. (2018) Neuro-, cardio-, and immunoplasticity: Effects of early adversity, *Annual Review of Psychology*, 69 (1), pp. 131–156.

Pan, W., Gao, X., Shi, S., Liu, F. and Li, C. (2018) Spontaneous brain activity did not show the effect of violent video games on aggression: A resting-state fMRI study, *Frontiers in Psychology*, 8 [online]. doi: 10.3389/fpsyg.2017.02219.

Panksepp, J. and Biven, L. (2012) *The Archaeology of Mind: Neuroevolutionary Origins of Human Emotion*. New York: Norton.

Park, B. Y., Wilson, G., Berger, J., Christman, M., Reina, B., Bishop, F., Klam, W. P. and Doan, A. P. (2016) Is internet pornography causing sexual dysfunctions? A review with clinical reports, *Behavioral Sciences*, 6 (3) [online]. doi: 10.3390/bs6030017.

Parnell, L., Felder, E., Prichard, H., Milstein, P. and Ewing, N. (2013) *Attachment-Focused EMDR: Healing Relational Trauma* (1st ed.). New York; London: W. W. Norton & Company.

Peake, P. K. (2017) Delay of gratification: Explorations of how and why children wait and its linkages to outcomes over the life course, in: Stevens, J. R. (ed.) *Impulsivity: How Time and Risk Influence Decision Making*. Cham: Springer, pp. 7–60.

Perry, B. D., Pollard, R. A., Blakley, T. L., Baker, W. L. and Vigilante, D. (1995) Childhood trauma, the neurobiology of adaptation, and 'use-dependent' development of the brain: How 'states' become 'traits', *Infant Mental Health Journal*, 16 (4), pp. 271–291.

Peterson, C., Maier, S. F. and Seligman, M. E. P. (1993) *Learned Helplessness: A Theory for the Age of Personal Control*. New York: Oxford University Press.

Piaget, J. (1965) *The Moral Judgement of the Child*. New York: Free Press.

Pinney, R., Schlachter, M. and Courtenay, A. (1983) *Bobby: Breakthrough of an Autistic Child*. London: Harvill.

Porges, S. W. (2011) *The Polyvagal Theory: Neurophysiological Foundations of Emotions, Attachment, Communication, and Self-Regulation*. New York: Norton.

Porto, J. A., Nunes, M. L. and Nelson, C. A. (2016) Behavioral and neural correlates of emotional development: Typically developing infants and infants of depressed and/or anxious mothers, *Journal de Pediatria*, 92 (3), pp. 14–22.

Provenzi, L., Casini, E., de Simone, P., Reni, G., Borgatti, R. and Montirosso, R. (2015) Mother–infant dyadic reparation and individual differences in vagal tone affect 4-month-old infants' social stress regulation, *Journal of Experimental Child Psychology*, 140, pp. 158–170.

Qiao, Y., Xie, B. and Du, X. (2012) Abnormal response to emotional stimulus in male adolescents with violent behavior in China, *European Child and Adolescent Psychiatry*, 21, pp. 193–198.

Rayner, E. (1991) *The Independent Mind in British Psychoanalysis*. New York: Jason Aronson.

Reddy, V. (2008) *How Infants Know Minds*. Cambridge, MA: Harvard University Press.

Reich, W. (1945) *Character Analysis*. New York: Farrar, Straus & Giroux.

Rey, H. and Magagna, J. E. (1994) *Universals of Psychoanalysis in the Treatment of Psychotic and Borderline States: Factors of Space-Time and Language*. London: Free Association Books.

Riser, D. K., Pegram, S. E. and Farley, J. P. (2013) Adolescent and young adult male sex offenders: Understanding the role of recidivism, *Journal of Child Sexual Abuse*, 22 (1), pp. 9–31.

Rizzolatti, G., Fogassi, L. and Gallese, V. (2006) Mirrors in the mind mirror neurons, a special class of cells in the brain, may mediate our ability to mimic, learn and understand the actions and intentions of others, *Scientific American*, 295 (5), pp. 54–61.

Roberts, J. A. and David, M. E. (2016) My life has become a major distraction from my cell phone: Partner phubbing and relationship satisfaction among romantic partners, *Computers in Human Behavior*, 54, pp. 134–141.

Roberts, J. A., Pullig, C. and Manolis, C. (2015) I need my smartphone: A hierarchical model of personality and cell-phone addiction, *Personality and Individual Differences*, 79, pp. 13–19.

Rogers, C. R. (1957) The necessary and sufficient conditions of therapeutic personality change, *Journal of Consulting Psychology*, 21 (2), pp. 240–248.

Rosenfeld, H. A. (1987) *Impasse and Interpretation: Therapeutic and Anti-Therapeutic Factors in the Psycho-Analytic Treatment of Psychotic, Borderline, and Neurotic Patients*. Oxford: Routledge.

Rudd, K. L., Alkon, A. and Yates, T. M. (2017) Prospective relations between intrusive parenting and child behavior problems: Differential moderation by parasympathetic nervous system regulation and child sex, *Physiology and Behavior*, 180, pp. 120–130.

Rutter, M., Andersen-Wood, L., Beckett, C., Bredenkamp, D., Castle, J., Groothues, C., Kreppner, J., Keaveney, L., Lord, C. and O'Connor, T. G. (1999)

Quasi-autistic patterns following severe early global privation, *Journal of Child Psychology and Psychiatry and Allied Disciplines*, 40 (4), pp. 537–549.

Safran, J. D., Muran, J. C. and Proskurov, B. (2009) Alliance, negotiation, and rupture resolution, in: Levy, R. A. and Ablon, J. S. (eds) *Handbook of Evidence-Based Psychodynamic Psychotherapy: Bridging the Gap between Science and Practice*. New York: Springer, pp. 201–225.

Sandler, J. (1993) On communication from patient to analyst: Not everything is projective identification, *International Journal of Psycho-Analysis*, 74, pp. 1097–1107.

Schaverien, J. (2015) *Boarding School Syndrome: The Psychological Trauma of the 'Privileged' Child*. Oxford: Routledge.

Schore, A. N. (1994) *Affect Regulation and the Origin of the Self: The Neurobiology of Emotional Development*. Hillsdale, NJ: Lawrence Erlbaum.

Schore, A. N. (2012) *The Science of the Art of Psychotherapy*. New York: Norton.

Sektnan, M., McClelland, M. M., Acock, A. and Morrison, F. J. (2010) Relations between early family risk, children's behavioral regulation, and academic achievement, *Early Childhood Research Quarterly*, 25 (4), pp. 464–479. doi: 10.1016/j.ecresq.2010.02.005.

Shai, D. and Belsky, J. (2017) Parental embodied mentalizing: How the nonverbal dance between parents and infants predicts children's socio-emotional functioning, *Attachment and Human Development*, 19 (2), pp. 191–219.

Shakespeare, W. (1914) *Macbeth*. Oxford: Oxford University Press.

Shedler, J. (2018) Where is the evidence for 'evidence-based' therapy? *Psychiatric Clinics of North America*, 41 (2), pp. 319–329.

Sheridan, M. A., Fox, N. A., Zeanah, C. H., McLaughlin, K. A. and Nelson, C. A. (2012) Variation in neural development as a result of exposure to institutionalization early in childhood, *Proceedings of the National Academy of Sciences*, 109 (32), pp. 12927–12932.

Shevrin, H., Smith, W. H. and Fitzler, D. E. (1971) Average evoked response and verbal correlates of unconscious mental processes, *Psychophysiology*, 8 (2), pp. 149–162.

Singer, T. and Klimecki, O. M. (2014) Empathy and compassion, *Current Biology*, 24 (18), pp. 875–878.

Sletvold, J. (2014) *The Embodied Analyst: From Freud and Reich to Relationality*. Oxford; New York: Routledge.

Sliwinski, J., Katsikitis, M. and Jones, C. M. (2017) A review of interactive technologies as support tools for the cultivation of mindfulness, *Mindfulness*, 8 (5), pp. 1150–1159.

Slutske, W. S., Moffitt, T. E., Poulton, R. and Caspi, A. (2012) Undercontrolled temperament at age 3 predicts disordered gambling at age 32: A longitudinal study of a complete birth cohort, *Psychological Science*, 23 (5), pp. 510–516.

Smith, C. E., Chen, D. and Harris, P. (2010) When the happy victimizer says sorry: Children's understanding of apology and emotion, *British Journal of Developmental Psychology*, 28 (Pt 4), pp. 727–746.

Smyke, A. T., Zeanah, C. H., Gleason, M. M., Drury, S. S., Fox, N. A., Nelson, C. A. and Guthrie, D. (2014) A randomized controlled trial comparing foster care and institutional care for children with signs of reactive attachment disorder, *American Journal of Psychiatry*, 169 (5), pp. 508–514.

Solms, M. and Panksepp, J. (2012) The 'id' knows more than the 'ego' admits: Neuropsychoanalytic and primal consciousness perspectives on the interface between affective and cognitive neuroscience, *Brain Sciences*, 2 (2), pp. 147–175.

Spitz, R. A. (1945) Hospitalism: An inquiry into the genesis of psychiatric conditions in early childhood, *Psychoanalytic Study of the Child*, 1, pp. 53–74.

Steiner, J. (1994) Patient-centered and analyst-centered interpretations: Some implications of containment and countertransference, *Psychoanalytic Inquiry*, 14 (3), pp. 406–422.

Stellar, J. E., Cohen, A., Oveis, C. and Keltner, D. (2015) Affective and physiological responses to the suffering of others: Compassion and vagal activity, *Journal of Personality and Social Psychology*, 108 (4), pp. 572–585.

Stern, D. N. (1985) *The Interpersonal World of the Infant*. New York: Basic Books.

Stipek, D. and Gralinski, J. H. (1996) Children's beliefs about intelligence and school performance, *Journal of Educational Psychology*, 88 (3), pp. 397–407.

Symington, N. (1983) The analyst's act of freedom as agent of therapeutic change, *International Review of Psycho-Analysis*, 10, pp. 283–291.

Symington, N. (1993) *Narcissism: A New Theory*. London: Karnac.

Teicher, M. H. and Samson, J. A. (2016) Annual research review: Enduring neurobiological effects of childhood abuse and neglect, *Journal of Child Psychology and Psychiatry*, 57 (3), pp. 241–266.

Teicher, M. H., Samson, J. A., Anderson, C. M. and Ohashi, K. (2016) The effects of childhood maltreatment on brain structure, function and connectivity, *Nature Reviews Neuroscience*, 17 (10), pp. 652–666.

Tizard, B. and Hodges, J. (1978) The effect of early institutional rearing on the development of 8-year-old children, *Journal of Child Psychology and Psychiatry*, 19 (2), pp. 99–118.

Tomasello, M. (2009) *Why We Cooperate*. Cambridge, MA: MIT Press.

Trevarthen, C. (2001) Intrinsic motives for companionship in understanding: Their origin, development, and significance for infant mental health, *Infant Mental Health Journal*, 22 (1–2), pp. 95–131.

Trevarthen, C. (2016) From the intrinsic motive pulse of infant actions to the lifetime of cultural meanings, in: Mölder, B., Arstila, V. and Øhrstrøm, P. (eds.) *Philosophy and Psychology of Time*. New York: Springer, pp. 225–265.

Trevarthen, C. and Hubley, P. (1978) Secondary intersubjectivity: Confidence, confiding and acts of meaning in the first year, in: Lock, A. (ed.) *Action, Gesture and Symbol: The Emergence of Language*. London: Academic Press, pp. 183–229.

Trivers, R. L. (1971) The evolution of reciprocal altruism, *Quarterly Review of Biology*, 46, pp. 35–57.

Tronick, E. (2007) *The Neurobehavioral and Social Emotional Development of Infants and Children*. New York: Norton.

Turkle, S. (2012) *Alone Together: Why We Expect More from Technology and Less from Each Other*. New York: Basic Books.

Tustin, F. (1992) *Autistic States in Children*. London: Tavistock.

van der Kolk, B. A. (2014) *The Body Keeps the Score*. London: Allen Lane.

Vanderwert, R. E., Zeanah, C. H., Fox, N. A. and Nelson, C. A. (2016) Normalization of EEG activity among previously institutionalized children placed into foster care: A 12-year follow-up of the Bucharest Early Intervention Project, *Developmental Cognitive Neuroscience*, 17, pp. 68–75.

Viding, E. and McCrory, E. J. (2018) Understanding the development of psychopathy: Progress and challenges, *Psychological Medicine*, 48 (4), pp. 566–577.

Voon, V. and Potenza, M. (2015) Compulsive sexual behaviour: The role of cue reactivity and attentional bias, *Journal of Behavioral Addictions*, 4 (S1), pp. 41–43.

Waller, R. and Hyde, L. W. (2018) Callous-unemotional behaviors in early childhood: The development of empathy and prosociality gone awry, *Current Opinion in Psychology*, 20, pp. 11–16.

Wampold, B. E. and Wampold, B. E. (2015) *The Great Psychotherapy Debate: Models, Methods, and Findings*. Oxford: Routledge.

Weierstall, R., Schalinski, I., Crombach, A., Hecker, T. and Elbert, T. (2012) When combat prevents PTSD symptoms: Results from a survey with former child soldiers in Northern Uganda, *BMC Psychiatry*, 12 (41), pp. 1–8.

Weierstall, R., Schauer, M. and Elbert, T. (2013) An appetite for aggression, *Scientific American Mind*, 24 (2), pp. 46–49.

Wiltermuth, S. S. and Heath, C. (2009) Synchrony and cooperation, *Psychological Science*, 20 (1), pp. 1–5.

Winnicott, D. W. (1953) *Through Paediatrics to Psycho-Analysis: Collected Papers*. New York: Basic Books.

Winnicott, D. W. (1965) *The Maturational Processes and the Facilitating Environment: Studies in the Theory of Emotional Development*. London: Hogarth Press.

Winnicott, D. W. (1971) *Playing and Reality*. New York: Basic Books.

Wood, H. (2013) Internet pornography and paedophilia, *Psychoanalytic Psychotherapy*, 27 (4), pp. 319–338.

Yakeley, J. (2009) *Working with Violence: A Contemporary Psychoanalytic Approach*. London: Palgrave Macmillan.

Zieber, N., Kangas, A., Hock, A. and Bhatt, R. S. (2014) Infants' perception of emotion from body movements, *Child Development*, 85 (2), pp. 675–684.

Zych, I., Baldry, A. C. and Farrington, D. P. (2017) School bullying and cyberbullying: Prevalence, characteristics, outcomes, and prevention, in: Hasselt, V. and Bourke, V. B. (eds.) *Handbook of Behavioral Criminology*. New York: Springer, pp. 113–138.

Index